THE GREAT PHYSICIAN'S

Rx

for

CHILDREN'S HEALTH

JORDAN RUBIN
with Fiona Blair, M.D.

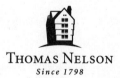

THOMAS NELSON
Since 1798

NASHVILLE   DALLAS   MEXICO CITY   RIO DE JANEIRO   BEIJING

Every effort has been made to make this book as accurate as possible. The purpose of this book is to educate. It is a review of scientific evidence that is presented for information purposes. No individual should use the information in this book for self-diagnosis, treatment, or justification in accepting or declining any medical therapy for any health problems or diseases. No individual is discouraged from seeking professional medical advice and treatment, and this book is not supplying medical advice. Any application of the information herein is at the reader's own discretion and risk. Therefore, any individual with a specific health problem or who is taking medications must first seek advice from his personal physician or health-care provider before starting a nutrition program. The author and Thomas Nelson Publishers, Inc., shall have neither liability nor responsibility to any person or entity with respect to loss, damage, or injury caused or alleged to be caused directly or indirectly by the information contained in this book. We assume no responsibility for errors, inaccuracies, omissions, or any inconsistency herein.

In view of the complex, individual nature of health and fitness problems, this book and the ideas, programs, procedures, and suggestions herein are not intended to replace the advice of trained medical professionals. All matters regarding one's health require medical supervision. A physician should be consulted prior to adopting any program or programs described in this book. The author and publisher disclaim any liability arising directly or indirectly from the use of this book.

Published in Nashville, Tennessee. Thomas Nelson is a trademark of Thomas Nelson, Inc.

Thomas Nelson, Inc. titles may be purchased in bulk for educational, business, fund-raising, or sales promotional use. For information, please e-mail SpecialMarkets@ThomasNelson.com.

Scripture quotations marked NKJV are taken from the NEW KING JAMES VERSION®. Copyright © 1979, 1980, 1982 by Thomas Nelson, Inc. Used by permission. All rights reserved.

Scripture quotations noted KJV are from the Holy Bible, KING JAMES VERSION.

Library of Congress Cataloging-in-Publication Data

Rubin, Jordan.
    The Great Physician's Rx for Children's Health / Jordan Rubin with Fiona Blair.
        p. cm.
ISBN 978-0-7852-1902-6
1. Self-care, Health.   2. Health.   I. Remedios, David.   II. Title.
    RA776.95.R828   2005
    613.2—dc22   2005024890

Printed in the United States of America

08 09 10 11 12 QW 5 4 3 2 1

To my beautiful son, Joshua Michael. May you grow up healthy and strong—physically, emotionally, mentally, and spiritually. I love you more than you'll ever know.

CONTENTS

INTRODUCTION

Offer Your Body as a Living Sacrifice

This was uncharted territory for us.

I had agreed to speak at a fund-raising event a couple of months earlier, figuring that since my expectant wife, Nicki, wasn't due to deliver our first child until June 5, 2004, it would be no problem for me to say a few words at this Friday evening event on Memorial Day Weekend.

The cause was a good one: Places of Hope International, a Christian humanitarian organization founded by Christ Fellowship in Palm Beach Gardens, Florida (where my family attends), was partnering with Biblical Health Institute, an organization I started in 2005, to put on a fund-raiser for its work in placing orphaned children with host families in nearby West Palm Beach.

After accepting the microphone that evening, I began by introducing my wife, whose bulging abdomen stuck out as only a pregnant woman's can in her ninth month of gestation. "If Nicki gets up and runs out of here, and you see me following her, you'll know why," I joked.

Then she felt a contraction—while I was speaking at the dedication dinner! Five or ten minutes later, another. At first she didn't say anything to her parents, who were seated with her, but by the time I had finished addressing the audience, we all realized that labor had officially begun.

"How far apart are your contractions?" asked her mom, a mother of three.

"I don't know," Nicki replied. "They're not real close together." So we didn't rush out of the auditorium. We got home at 10 p.m.

We tried to get some rest, but Nicki's contractions were becoming more frequent and were increasing in intensity. Finally, exhausted from a lack of sleep, I called our midwife, Ally, at the ungodly hour of 4 a.m. (We had chosen to use a nurse/midwife who delivered babies in hospitals. That way, if there were complications, trained medical staff were just steps away.)

After listening to my breathless, before-dawn report, Ally said, "It sounds like we have some time. I'll meet you at the Jupiter Medical Center in an hour." This was our local hospital, whose slogan was, "Men are from Mars, but babies are from Jupiter."

We checked into Birthing Room #1 shortly after 5 a.m. Next door, in Room #2, was our close friend Denise Duke, who had given birth to a baby girl, Aubrey, on Friday morning. Talk about a coincidence only the Lord could have orchestrated: Denise had suffered three miscarriages before becoming pregnant with Aubrey. Not twenty-four hours earlier, I had visited Denise and her husband, Kenny (a childhood friend), and played cootchie-coo with baby Aubrey, so I had a strong sense of déjà vu.

Another coincidence was the fact that, like Denise, Nicki's road to childbirth was also difficult: She had been trying to conceive for two and a half years. We were nearly resigned to being an infertile couple when my wife miraculously became pregnant. In fact, Nicki and Denise had both become pregnant after following a forty-day diet and lifestyle plan that I created for my book *The Maker's Diet*.

The fact that the Lord would put our two families next door to each other was beyond coincidence to me. Still, I knew better than to knock on Denise's door at 5:30 a.m. the day after she delivered a baby. Besides, the more pressing concern was determining how far along Nicki was. Ally measured her at seven centimeters dilated. When Nicki's water broke minutes later, we thought things would soon sail along as nature intended.

Not much happened, though. I couldn't kill time fast enough to share the exciting developments with Denise. I waited all the way until 7 a.m. before dropping by to see if mother and child were doing well in Room #2. Denise was awake and was just as surprised to see me as I was overjoyed to visit her.

But when I returned to Nicki, our midwife told us that her labor was not progressing the way it should. At that point, the doula[1] that we had also hired began massaging Nicki's legs and arms as I encouraged and prayed for her. Because she wanted to go as far as possible without medication, Nicki didn't opt for an epidural or an infusion of Pitocin to move labor along. But as the contractions lumbered into the early afternoon hours without any significant progress, we decided that enough was enough.

Poor Nicki. Even with Pitocin circulating in her bloodstream, nothing happened. As she pushed and pushed, her face swelled, and her eyes got puffy from the heroic exertions. I stroked her matted hair while the doula worked her magic fingers, but it was distressing to see my wife suffering such intense pain hour after hour. In fact, her screams could be heard in the hallway by our worried parents.

Finally, at 6 p.m., after twenty hours of agony, she managed to push Joshua Michael Rubin into the world. Everything changed the moment he drew a breath and cried his lungs out. I felt an overwhelming sense of love as well as a sober responsibility to father an innocent child who had his entire life ahead of him.

At first, I wasn't sure how to hold Joshua because I was afraid he was so delicate. But as I rocked him in my arms and our eyes met for the first time, I repeated my resolve to raise him to be the healthiest boy possible. After all, his newborn body was a blank slate, pure and uncontaminated by fast food, soda pop, candy bars, and other junk foods. His incredible immune system hadn't been battered by allergies, viruses, and parasites, and he had not yet been exposed to environmental toxins such as chlorinated water and pesticides in his food. His infant body was just waiting to grow up big and strong.

On the morning of May 29, 2004, I solemnly promised before God that I would raise Joshua to the best of my abilities. This book will describe how that journey has gone so far, and I will also share ways that you can raise your children according to the principles of the Great Physician's prescription for health and wellness.

Joshua is three years old as I write this, and to the best of my knowledge, he hasn't eaten any:

- processed foods
- pasteurized, homogenized dairy products from animals injected with hormones and antibiotics
- commercially produced meat from grain-fed cattle
- white sugar or table salt

In other words, Joshua hasn't swallowed anything that man conjured up in a laboratory. Instead, my son has consumed nothing but foods that God created in a form healthy for his body, thanks to our around-the-clock effort to nourish our little guy with a 100 percent, all-natural, beyond-organic diet. I think the worst thing we've ever fed him during his infancy was store-bought organic sweet potatoes from a jar.

So how's he doing?

Thanks for asking. If you've got a minute, I have some photos here in my wallet . . .

Seriously, although Joshua was born with fairly normal height and weight measurements (7 pounds, 10 ounces and 21½ inches), our pediatrician says that today Joshua ranks in the 90th to 95th percentile in height and weight and is on schedule to grow up "big and strong." Don't get the idea that he's a candidate for childhood obesity; there's no lingering baby fat on his pint-sized hard body. He's a robust, energetic toddler who's a Tasmanian devil around the house. He's really never been laid low by a flu bug or serious head cold, and if his nose sniffles a bit, he's fine the next day.

Joshua has yet to be administered an antibiotic and has had few tummy aches, allergies, or signs of asthma. He's also managed to avoid ear infections, which other parents tell me is a minor miracle these days. His only doctor visits, other than well baby appointments, were for a busted lip and a chicken pox–like rash.

I recognize that describing Joshua's excellent health at three years of age is a little like a football coach boasting about a 14-0 lead early in the first quarter.

Please know that both Nicki and I recognize that there's still a lot of game to be played. In fact, we're anticipating plenty of challenges ahead, or "adversity," as football coaches call it.

But at this time in his young life, Joshua's making all the right plays. He loves salad, as well as veggies like broccoli, peppers, zucchini, and carrots. He's keen on grass-fed buffalo, venison, and wild-caught fish. He devours fresh fruit by the bowlful. And he can't get enough sheep's milk yogurt. We're also amazed at what Joshua *won't* eat. We've seen him shake his head when offered cake, cookies, lollipops, and all sorts of candy. Even at his tender age, he *knows* what isn't healthy for him.

What about your children? Do they have winning health, or have they fallen behind in the score? Are you pleased with their weight and fitness, or have they given up a couple of touchdowns? You're their health coach, the person responsible for their well-being, so they're depending on you.

If you've been bewildered by all the parenting advice on how to raise children in the healthiest possible manner, let *The Great Physician's Rx for Children's Health* be your playbook. In upcoming chapters, I'll be sharing seven keys to health and wellness that will unlock your children's health potential and give you the tools you need to raise those kids you love more than anything in the world. I'm asking you to incorporate these timeless principles into your children's lives and allow God to transform their health physically, mentally, emotionally, and spiritually.

Whom Does This Book Target?

In *The Great Physician's Rx for Children's Health*, I'll be relating the seven keys to health and wellness for children between infancy and adolescence—in other words, children ages 0 to 12. I hope to write a book on teen health sometime in the future.

Living by Her Rules

My generation grew up with Miss Piggy, the porky puppet who made her first appearance on *The Muppet Show* in 1976, the year after I was born. "I always knew I was destined for *le* top," she once told *TV Guide*.

Miss Piggy's queen-sized snout and ample figure belied a self-confidence born out of the self-esteem movement that picked up steam in the 1970s. When the *New York Times* asked her if fame had changed her, she haughtily replied, "I am still just little *Moi*, the same gorgeous and supremely talented pig. Beauty is my curse." Like I said, Miss Piggy was not lacking in self-confidence.

The glamorous Miss Piggy proclaimed to live by three rules:

1. Eat what you want.

2. Exercise your prerogative.

3. Find a good plastic surgeon who gives frequent-flyer miles.[2]

The Heavy Burden of Stereotyping

Parents say they want their children to grow up to be doctors, firefighters, or cowboys—anything but fat. That's because society has a built-in bias against the obese, and that attitude carries over to the job market.

A number of studies have documented that heavyset adults earn less than those who are thin. Overly fat people are routinely stereotyped as lazy, slow, and unmotivated as compared with those at a healthier weight, who are more likely to be described as smart, competent, and attractive.[3]

Even overweight people prefer to be around thin people, according to *Obesity Research* magazine.[4]

Kids loved her saucy attitude, and adults caught the inside jokes, but if a real-life Miss Piggy attended elementary school today, she would secretly wish she was a pound of bacon for all the verbal abuse she would endure during recess. Kids say the cruelest things, and those with weight problems are sitting ducks for subtle jibes and mean names like "Fatso," "Blimpie," "Blubber," "Porker," "Thunder Thighs," or "Lard Butt." And woe to the heavyset girl named Patty or Tina because she'll get tagged as "Fatty Patty" or "Tubby Tina." Boys love re-creating fat jokes they've viewed over and over on movies like *Shallow Hal* and *The Nutty Professor*.

These days there isn't a lack of targets in the schoolyard because of a massive wave that has hit our shoreline like a tsunami—childhood obesity. This is not to excuse the present cohort of American adults, who are fatter, less fit, and more prone to disease than previous generations. But today's younger generation is supersized as never before in human history. And it's all happened in the last twenty-five years!

Over the past few decades, a steady but dramatic increase in obesity has occurred throughout the entire US population, but nowhere has this been more noticeable than among our children. Currently, one-third of America's youth are either obese or at risk of becoming obese. Over the past thirty years, the obesity rate has nearly *tripled* (from 5 to 14 percent) for children ages two to five and *quadrupled* (from 5 percent to 19 percent) for children ages six to eleven, according to a report from the Institute of Medicine.[5] Overall, the number of obese children is expected to rise to one in five, or 20 percent, by 2010, prompting Richard H. Carmona, M.D., the US surgeon general from 2002 to 2006, to declare, "Generation Y is turning into Generation XL."[6]

I know that one's eyes start to glaze over after a couple of sentences of statistics, so let me insert a paragraph from a column written by *Sports Illustrated*'s Rick Reilly that pretty much sums things up on the child obesity front:

> Is your Little Leaguer so fat his blood type is Chee-tos? Do the other kids wait for your Cub Scout to jump in the pool so they can ride the wave? Is it difficult

for your six-year-old to play Hide and Seek anymore? *I see you, Amber! At both ends of the Buick!*

Chubby girls are now singing this rope-skipping rhyme:

Georgia, Texas
North Carolina!
I think I'm suff-ring
Acute angina![7]

Trade Deficit

Chinese exports fill our kids' closets with clothes, shoes, and plastic toys, but we're exporting a dubious commodity in return: childhood obesity.

China, the world's most populous country, has struggled to feed the masses enough rice for centuries. In the last twenty years, though, economic expansion has produced higher standards of living, resulting in more discretionary *yuan* for packaged foods and trips to McDonald's and Kentucky Fried Chicken.

Mickey D's and KFC in China? You betcha. There are hundreds of them there, and the Chinese have gone gaga over Big Macs and crispy fried chicken from the Colonel. The introduction of fast food, plus more sedentary lifestyles and video games, has resulted in a supersizing of Chinese children. The Chinese Health Ministry announced that urban Chinese boys were 2.5 inches taller and 6.6 pounds heavier than they were thirty years ago.[9] Eight percent of ten- to twelve-year-olds in Chinese cities are considered obese, and another 15 percent are overweight. Sadly, bigger children are viewed in their culture as proof of prosperity, as evidenced by an old saying: "A fat child is a healthy child."

It will take some time for attitudes to change, but I just wish the Chinese knew that our fast-food exports have a bigger price tag than their manufactured goods.

After reading this, you're either chuckling or really ticked at the insensitivity, but it's no laughing matter when it's *your* kid who could be euphemistically described as "big-boned" or "husky." Childhood obesity has become a national topic in conversation because parents are waking up to the fact that their children's extra pounds today put them at risk for significant health problems tomorrow. A body of research has found that obese kids are likely—a 79 percent probability, according to one study[8]—to become overweight adults who'll live lower-quality lives that could result in their early, untimely deaths.

If you're hoping that your son will "grow out" of his chubbiness, you need to take off your rose-colored glasses. "Contrary to popular belief, young children who are overweight or obese typically won't lose the extra weight simply as a result of getting older," said Duane Alexander, M.D., the director of NIH's National Institute of Child Health and Human Development.[10]

The unblinking reality is that overweight and obese children face considerable heath perils in the future, including these serious diseases:

- **Type 2 diabetes:** If there was ever a black cloud hanging over the horizon, it's type 2 diabetes, which has become a growing concern in the last decade since it can cause blindness, heart and kidney disease, and loss of limbs. Unfortunately, the number of prescriptions for the treatment or prevention of type 2 diabetes in children doubled between 2001 and 2005.[11]

  By definition, diabetes is a chronic degenerative disease caused by the body's inability to either produce enough insulin or properly use insulin, which is essential for the proper metabolism of blood sugar, also known as glucose. (For those of you who last heard about insulin back in high school biology class, insulin is a hormone the body uses to convert sugar, starches, and other foods into energy for the cells.)

  Type 2 diabetes, the most common form of diabetes, is difficult to diagnose and challenging to treat with modern medicine techniques.

With type 2 diabetes, the pancreas either does not produce enough insulin, or the cells ignore the insulin produced by the body. Since insulin regulates and maintains the body's circulation of sugar levels, the body's inability to metabolize blood sugar—for whatever reason—opens the door to a host of medical complications including kidney failure, eye problems possibly leading to blindness, tooth and gum infections, and circulation blockages that cause heart disease or heart attacks.

The Centers for Disease Control (CDC) predicts that one out of three children born after the year 2000 will eventually develop type 2 diabetes. Furthermore, researchers say those who develop type 2 diabetes before the age of fifteen will have a shortened life expectancy of approximately *fifteen* years.[12] That's why some demographers are worried that Joshua's generation could live fewer years than today's life expectancy, which is 75.2 years for men and 80.4 years for women, according to the National Center for Health Statistics.[13]

- **High cholesterol and high blood pressure:** An estimated 61 percent of overweight young people face at least one additional risk factor for heart disease, such as high cholesterol or high blood pressure.[14] Elevated cholesterol levels cause the development of cholesterol-containing fatty deposits—known as plaque—to form and begin traveling through the blood vessels. Over time, plaque clogs arteries and veins, like sludge in a drainpipe. The earlier that plaque develops in young blood vessels, the worse for the body.

   High blood pressure—also known as hypertension—increases one's risk of developing cardiovascular disease or kidney disease, as well as having a stroke. The scary thing about high blood pressure is that there are no warning signs or symptoms for this condition, which is why it has been nicknamed the "silent killer." Significantly elevated blood pressure has been found more commonly in obese children than in their non-obese peers.[15]

- **Pediatric GERD:** Doctors are seeing more cases of pediatric gastroe-sophageal reflux disease, which is much more painful than a regular stomachache. To show you how new pediatric GERD is, the oldest support organization, Pediatric/Adolescent Gastroesophageal Reflux Association, was formed in 1992.

- **Joint stress:** The weight-bearing joints of obese kids—hips, knees, and ankles—aren't designed to survive the additional pounding that comes from hefting excess weight. Degenerative arthritis of the hips, knees, and ankles is inevitable and limits physical activity, which sets in motion a vicious circle: more weight, more pain, and less activity.

    At a time when young bodies are growing like weeds, obesity can lead to bowing of the legs and the possibility of more bone fractures. Obesity researcher Jack Yanovski found that overweight children were far more likely to suffer a fracture than their ideal-weight peers. Heavy children also had more bone and hip joint abnormalities, which can lead to permanent deformities.[16]

    As children become young adults, sharp pain and swollen, tender joints, as well as stiff spines, creaky necks, and bad backs, can sap vitality from their lives at a time when they should be at their physical peaks.

- **Other risks:** Not to pile on, but other health dangers include shortness of breath and/or asthma, sleep apnea, skin rashes, and clinical depres-sion. Obesity has been long associated with low self-esteem.

    Looking to the future, too many children born since 2000 will need insulin injections, experience kidney problems, live with weakened immune systems, go on liver dialysis, and battle glaucoma and other eye problems related to diabetes.

The Root Causes

Why are our kids in this mess?

It's easy to play the blame game. Kids learn quickly which buttons to push to effectively provoke parents to purchase sugar-frosted cereals, glazed doughnuts, and fried chicken that's finger-lickin' good. Billion-dollar food companies heavily advertise their sweet cereals and salty snacks on kid-friendly channels like Nickelodeon and the Cartoon Network, trying to hook young children as life-long customers. School districts around the country have canceled PE classes or curtailed energetic recess games like tag for bocce ball or, as Rick Reilly wrote, "competitive cup-stacking."[17] Xbox and PlayStation video games capture millions of young eyeballs during the after-school hours. The only other part of their owners' anatomies getting exercised is their thumbs.

I'm sure we could come up with a dozen more reasons why childhood obesity has become a nationwide epidemic, but in my view, everything boils down to two words: *parental control.*

Please understand I'm generalizing here, but when you look at the big picture, too many fathers and mothers have lost command of the parental ship. They are:

- unwilling to say no to their kids' demands for junk food;
- unmotivated to cook and prepare meals from fresh fruits, vegetables, whole grains, and meats;
- uneducated about the importance of nutritional supplementation;
- unaccustomed to exercising regularly;
- unaware that they and their children are living in a toxic world;
- uninformed about deadly emotions; and
- unprepared to teach their children to live lives of prayer and purpose.

Two scenes that are burned into my memory happened on the way back from a trip to Pennsylvania. At the airport departure gate, I witnessed a young mother handing her approximately eighteen-month-old toddler one McDonald's French fry after another. Not one hour later, while seated on the airplane, I saw another young mother grinning at the person seated next to her as her four-month-old infant sat on her lap and sipped a dark cola—probably Coke—from her cup.

What were those mothers thinking? After my initial shock, I felt bummed by what I saw. *The poor kids*, I thought. What they ate and drank bordered on child abuse. Then I recalled a verse of Scripture that I often share when I speak to churches on Sunday morning. "My people are destroyed for lack of knowledge," says Hosea 4:6 (NJKV). Those young moms were probably unmindful that they were harming their children by feeding them unhealthy fried foods and sugary beverages. Or maybe they did know but didn't care.

I understand that what I've written may sound judgmental, even harsh. I'm sure parents with older kids are smirking right about now: *Just wait, Jordan, until Joshua gets a little older*, you may be thinking. *Then you'll see how tough it is to be a parent.*

I'm sure we'll have our difficult and painful moments, but the verse I'm holding on to is Proverbs 22:6, which is God's Word on how to exercise parental leadership: "Train up a child in the way he should go, and when he is old he will not depart from it" (NKJV).

The first word in the sentence, the Hebrew word *hanak*, doesn't actually mean "train up," but, according to the *Theological Wordbook of the Old Testament*, indicates a meaning closer to "inaugurate," "initiate," "begin," or "start off."[18] James A. Fowler of Christ in You Ministries says that the next phrase—"in the way he should go"—is derived from two Hebrew words: The first, *peh*, literally means "mouth" but figuratively refers to an "opening" or "entrance." The second Hebrew word, *derek*, literally means "road" or "pathway" but refers figuratively to a journey, course, or way.[19]

Start off a child at the entrance to the journey of life . . . now, that adds a new layer of meaning to this verse. What the Lord is saying through King Solomon's proverb is that it's your responsibility to guide your children through the preliminaries of life, right from the beginning, because lifetime habits are formed during childhood. "What happens before the age of two has a permanent, lasting effect on your health," said Dr. David J. P. Barker, a professor of medicine at Oregon Health and Science University in Portland, Oregon.[20]

Growing Up in the Rubin Home

You may be wondering, *What kind of home did you grow up in, Jordan? What did your parents teach you about healthy living?*

My parents, Herb and Phyllis Rubin, have long been health conscious. They got into natural and organic foods in the early 1970s, but for them, unlike many of their peers in the Baby Boom generation, eating healthfully was not a fad. They viewed processed foods or anything with preservatives as poison.

This was an early reaction—rebellion, actually—to all the "synthetic food" being foisted on a gullible public in the '60s. The Mercury Seven astronauts (including Alan Shepard, John Glenn, and Gus Grissom) drank a water-and-orange-powder concoction called Tang while they circled the globe. A popular Saturday morning cartoon show, *The Jetsons*, showed the futuristic family eating meals in capsule form. Food technologists created other foods in the laboratory and heavily marketed them: Carnation Instant Breakfast, Pop-Tarts, Kool-Aid, Cool Whip, chicken pot pies, frozen pizza, and a whole slew of baked goods derived from bleached flour and loaded with shelf-friendly preservatives. Other examples are Wonder Bread, Ding Dongs, and Twinkies.

My parents were among the first to turn their backs on all that "plastic food." Their motto was, "The more natural, the better," and they filled their cupboards with raw honey, wheat germ, and granola and their refrigerator with farm-fresh organic fruits and vegetables. Not only did they adopt the back-to-nature lifestyle (as it was called back then), but my father also promoted it wholeheartedly at his work. He became a naturopathic physician and chiropractor who employed a more natural approach to treating patients who saw him for a variety of aches and pains.

Most importantly, though, Mom and Dad raised me according to the Bible. Yes, Rubin is a Jewish surname, and my family is Jewish, and my parents became Messianic Jews when they put their faith and hope in Yeshua (Jesus) as their Messiah when I was two years old. I remember, when I was entering kindergarten, believing that Jesus came to earth and died for my sins. I've been a believer ever since.

As their firstborn child (a sister, Jenna, would arrive four years and nine months later), Mom and Dad raised me with natural and organic foods. I didn't eat any meat the first four years of my life, but then my parents decided that I needed the important nutrients from chicken and fish in my diet. Kids in my neighborhood didn't exactly flock to our house after school because Mom banned Lay's potato chips, Oreos, and Fudgsicles. But if they wanted a wheat-grass smoothie or some home-made granola, they came to the right place.

While I ate very well at home, whenever I went to school or my friends' homes, I scarfed down the junk food. Maybe it was the "forbidden fruit" syndrome. During school lunch, I can remember trying to trade baby carrots for corn chips or cookies but not finding many takers. Some of my classmates, however, were willing to part with some of their Laffy Taffy or Milk Duds for a quarter, so I took them up on their generous offers.

It wasn't until my body was attacked by chronic digestive and immune system diseases that left me at death's door at the age of nineteen that I stopped eating junk food and looked to the Bible as a single, constant source for health and wellness. For the rest of my story, you'll have to read one of my previous books, *The Maker's Diet* or *The Great Physician's Rx for Health and Wellness.*

I believe the first two years of life are as crucial as it gets when it comes to good health, and that's why Nicki and I went the extra mile to feed Joshua only foods made from the purest, most organic sources and to never use the microwave to heat his homemade infant formula. (I'll have more to say about microwave ovens in Key #5, "Reduce Toxins in Their Environment.")

There is no better or more important resource in this world than our children. We hear that said a lot, but once you become a parent, that commonplace expression takes on a whole new meaning. I would imagine that millions of older parents, looking at their unhealthy adult sons and daughters in their thirties and forties, wish they could go back in time and do it all over again. "Experience: that most brutal of teachers," said C. S. Lewis, author of *The Chronicles of Narnia.* "But you learn. My God, do you learn."

My heart's desire is that you will embrace the prescription from the Great Physician and pass it along to those children—whether by virtue of birth or

---

What Type of Parent Are You?

Your parenting style has a big impact on your child's weight, according to a National Institute of Child Health and Human Development study.[21] Children of authoritarian parents had five times the risk of being overweight compared to children of *authoritative* parents.

What's the difference between authoritarian and authoritative parents? Authoritarian parents will demand that their preschoolers finish every vegetable on their plate, for instance, while authoritative parents would offer a couple of different vegetables and allow the child to decide which one he wants to eat.

The researchers evaluated two other parenting styles: permissive, in which indulgent parents don't practice discipline in the home; and neglectful, in which uninvolved parents don't set any rules. Parents of permissive and neglectful mothers were twice as likely to be overweight as children of authoritative mothers.

Authoritative parents maintain boundaries and teach their children good eating habits, which, to me, is what Proverbs 22:6 is all about.

adoption—who will live beyond you. Although Nicki and I have learned a great deal in three short years with Joshua, we understand that doesn't make us experts in child raising, but it has allowed us to put into practice the principles behind the Great Physician's prescription for health and wellness. Just as we've experienced major health transformations in our own lives, Nicki and I have witnessed outstanding health in not only our son, but also those who've responded to my message of health after reading one of my books or hearing me speak.

Perhaps you've just begun treading the road of raising those children whom God entrusted you with. Maybe a young one is on the way, or perhaps your quiver is full and you're just trying to raise the healthiest kids you can. No matter what your family situation is, adopting the *Great Physician's Rx for Children's Health* will give your impressionable sons and daughters their best chance to stay away from type 2 diabetes, high cholesterol, high blood pressure, acid reflux, severe joint pain, and ill health.

The Great Physician's Rx for Children's Health isn't about producing the best-looking, most athletic, or most charming kids in the history of the human race; it's about adding healthy years to your children's lives—years in which they can be at their physical, emotional, and spiritual best. I can think of no greater legacy for a parent.

The fact that you're holding this book means that this topic resonates with you. What I'm hoping is that the Great Physician's Rx for Children's Health will equip you to raise the healthiest children possible because, if I can turn an old phrase, an ounce of child raising is worth far more than a ton of cure when they become adults. My approach is based on seven keys to unlocking your children's health potential—a variation on principles that were established in my foundational book, *The Great Physician's Rx for Health and Wellness*.

The seven keys are:

Key #1: Teach Them to Eat to Live

Key #2: Supplement Their Diets with Whole Food Nutritional
Supplements

Key #3: Introduce Your Children to Advanced Hygiene

Key #4: Condition Their Bodies with Exercise and Body Therapies

Key #5: Reduce Toxins in Their Environment

Key #6: Help Them Avoid Deadly Emotions

Key #7: Lead Them to Live a Life of Prayer and Purpose

Some of the ideas I share in the coming chapters will come across as radical. Others will sound like common sense. But if you're looking for a plan to help your children finish the race that God intended for their lives, why not take a prescription from the Great Physician, the One who knew your children while they were still in the womb, the One who has plans to prosper them and not to harm them, to give them a great future and a hope (see Jeremiah 29:11).

INTRODUCING FIONA BLAIR, M.D.

A note from Jordan Rubin:

Although I consider myself well versed in naturopathic medicine, nutrition, and fitness, I lack the conventional medical background or hands-on experience of treating babies and youngsters in pediatric health. That's why I've asked Fiona Blair, M.D., a Harvard- and Emory University–trained pediatrician from Atlanta, to partner with me in the writing of The Great Physician's Rx for Children's Health.

Dr. Blair has an oversized heart for treating heavyset children whose poor nutrition and minimal exercise have contributed to a variety of ills. She's appeared numerous times on CNN's Headline News as a medical expert whenever the topic of childhood obesity makes the news, which, unfortunately, is quite often these days. You'll be reading her insights about children's health throughout this book, but I want you to get to know this remarkable person here first:

I was born in England in 1966 to Jamaican parents who immigrated to Massachusetts when I was three years old. My father was a pastor in the Pentecostal church, and my mother was a labor and delivery nurse, which sparked my interest in medicine, since I hung around hospitals during my early years.

When I was ten years old, however, Mom died of ovarian cancer, leaving behind a grieving husband and two daughters—myself and my sister, Simone. Three years later, we moved to Atlanta, where Dad was elevated to Bishop in the Church of God denomination. With a father as a pastor, I've always had the church as the core of my life, including singing and being involved in the worship part of the service.

Meanwhile, I became a very active student at Southwest DeKalb High School in Decatur, an Atlanta suburb. I was part of the student council, belonged to the drama club, and competed in talent shows. DeKalb was a racially mixed high school, and I belonged to all groups and never had my own clique. I was popular in the sense that people knew me, which explains why my classmates voted me homecoming queen my senior year. Looking back, I didn't feel beautiful growing up because beauty was defined a certain way in the popular culture, and I didn't think I fit that mold.

In a class of three hundred seniors at DeKalb, I graduated first in my class, which opened up all sorts of possibilities. When I told my guidance counselor that Harvard University was my number-one choice, she said, "You cannot be serious." I was serious, though, and when my acceptance came though, I was thrilled to return to Massachusetts, which felt a bit like home since I had lived there for ten years.

I was a psychology major and pre-med at Harvard, but during my four years of undergraduate work, I always knew I wanted to become a doctor. Following graduation, I took a year off to do some gospel singing while I applied to various medical schools. During that sabbatical, I met a handsome young man—Everton Lloyd Blair. We fell in love and got engaged. Meanwhile, Temple University accepted me into their medical school, but after completing a year at Temple, I transferred to Emory University in Atlanta because I was getting married to Everton, who was starting his career in information technology.

What a hectic time in my life! In the early 1990s, I was going to medical school, followed by a three-year residency program for pediatrics. My first child, Everton Lloyd II—nicknamed EJ for Everton Junior—arrived during my third year of medical school, and then Justin joined us during my second year of residency. Talk about a juggling act! The only way I survived was through the support of my husband as well as family members who lived close by, including my dad and my new mom (Dad remarried after my mother's death, and they had two children, Gregory and Brenton), my sister, and my aunts and uncles. The joke in my family is that everyone has babysat the children at one time or another.

Following my internship, I joined the Sulton Pediatric Group in 1996, where I worked diligently for ten years and built up quite a clientele. During this time, I also brought two more children into the world: Courtney and Brandon. Then in 2006, I decided to leave Sulton Pediatric and start my own practice, the ABC Pediatric Group in Stone Mountain, Georgia, *and* become an ordained minister to serve at our church, Bride Temple Church. These days I'm the praise team leader and choir director, playing the piano and organ while singing.

But enough about me. The reason I'm excited to assist Jordan is because of my passion for children's health. As a pediatrician who treats dozens of less-than-healthy children each day, I'm on the front lines of the childhood obesity epidemic, which is ravaging their health. I am seeing things in ten-year-old children that I don't like to see: type 2 diabetes, hypertension, and cardiovascular disease. It breaks my heart because these are medical conditions that these poor kids will have to deal with for the next sixty or seventy years, if they live that long ... and some won't. Either way, we're talking decades of seeing doctors routinely, taking medications, and dealing with a decrease in their quality of life.

The unfortunate thing about modern medicine is that I don't have time to sit and counsel patients. Many times, I wish I had forty-five minutes or an hour to educate parents and their children about how to eat right or the importance of after-school exercise, but HMOs and insurance companies will not pay for that. An op-ed piece in the *New York Times*, entitled "The Doctor Will See You for Exactly Seven Minutes," pretty much sums up where health care is these days.[22]

This is why *The Great Physician's Rx for Children's Health* is so important. I can't wait to hand this book to moms and dads looking for answers to their children's health care problems. Jordan's seven keys line up well with my holistic approach to medicine, and they are principles that I practice with my own children.

I believe that by the time you finish reading *The Great Physician's Rx for Children's Health*, you will be educated on the steps you can take to raise vibrant and healthy kids.

KEY #1

Teach Them to Eat to Live

I clutched Joshua, dressed in his best play clothes, in the crook of my left arm as Nicki and I entered the beautifully decorated home covered in pink crepe paper and helium balloons. One of Joshua's classmates from preschool, a cutie whom I'll call Caitlin, was celebrating her third birthday.

Boy, was Joshua excited to be there! This was his *first* "invited-to" birthday party, and something about the pink party decorations and the "hot air balloons," as he called them, told him that this afternoon's fiesta was a big deal. I set Joshua down and watched him pedal his tiny feet toward his preschool chums with an elated grin on his face.

Then Joshua eyed a bowl of colorful M&M candies perched on an end table next to the living room couch. I intercepted him just as he gathered his first handful. "No, Joshua. These are candy, and candy isn't good for you," I reminded him, picking up my son to distract him. The other parents, however, weren't concerned in the slightest when their children grabbed M&Ms—as well as potato chips and pretzels—by the fistful, along with their favorite flavor of boxed juice drinks.

A half hour later, the Domino's driver arrived bearing boxes of warm pizza. While the kids and adults attacked the pepperoni-and-cheese pies, heavy on the grease and high in calories, Joshua was content to eat the snacks we had brought along for him. He also grazed on the sliced carrots, purple grapes, and ruby red strawberries set out for the "adults" to eat. I remember thinking, *Why would parents assume that their kids wouldn't eat healthy foods at a birthday party?*

After Caitlin made her wish and blew out three candles, the party began breaking up. Upon departure, every child received a lovely parting gift—a Batman bag bulging with Tootsie Rolls, lollipops, fruit-flavored Starbursts, Trident gum, Nerd Ropes, Hot Tamales, and Gummy Body Parts candy, which are chewable confections in the grotesque forms of tongues, noses, fingers, teeth, and eyeballs.

Nicki and I accepted Joshua's Batman bag on his behalf, politely thanked the hosts, and dropped the sack of candy into the trash the minute we arrived home. Were we bothered by the goodie bag or the unhealthy foods set out at a birthday party attended by mostly two- and three-year-olds? Well, we were certainly disappointed, but since Nicki and I live in the real world, we realize that is how many families live and eat.

The day after Caitlin's birthday party, I accompanied Joshua to the Palm Beach Zoo, where we stopped by the baby monkey exhibit. Joshua was greatly amused by the antics of the little critters, but what struck me was a prominent sign attached to the enclosure:

> Please DO NOT feed us.
> We are on special diets.
> Your snacks make us sick.

I shook my head at the irony. Parents who wouldn't dream of feeding innocent baby monkeys a handful of popcorn, potato chips, or M&Ms—because it would have been unhealthy for these primates—have no problem setting out sweet-and-salty junk for their children to munch on.

We Deserve a Break Today

Nicki and I know that Joshua will be invited to many more birthday parties in the future, including invitations requesting his presence at a local McDonald's with an enclosed PlayPlace. Since we would never take Joshua to the Golden Arches, how will we handle that sticky situation?

We've talked about this, and one thing Nicki and I agree on is that we will not adopt a holier-than-thou attitude with the parents of Joshua's friends, sending vibes that we're too good to be seen at fast-food places or to eat their lousy food. Saying things like, "I wouldn't let my kids near that McDonald's junk in a million years," won't win hearts or minds to the Great Physician's prescription.

We will explain to the party hosts that, yes, Joshua would love to come, but he'll be bringing his own snacks. If they ask why, we'll describe how we've been steering our son away from fast food because it's unhealthy to eat. If that prompts a healthy discussion regarding the merits of Big Macs or the levels of trans fat found in McDonald's fries, then so be it. (McDonald's plans to switch to a trans fat–free vegetable oil blend in early 2008, but the shoestring potatoes will still be fried in unhealthy oils.)

Our goal has been to satisfy Joshua with such fantastic foods at home that he'll never have the desire to try a Big Mac or sample McDonald's iconic fries. Ever since he was an infant, we've done our best to explain—in age-appropriate language—why fast-food cheeseburgers, greasy fries, and hot fudge sundaes (unless Daddy makes them at home, which I've been known to do, by the way) don't meet the family standard.

So if Joshua gets invited to a play date at McDonald's, he'll be allowed to dive into a pool of plastic balls with his friends, but we will insist that he eat something at home first before we drop him off with some fruit-and-veggie snacks in his small backpack. We're confident he'll say no to sharing a friend's Happy Meal.

I wonder how much good these warnings do, however. I contend that very few parents today *really* understand how absolutely detrimental the standard

American diet is to their children's health because if they did, we wouldn't have a national health crisis on our hands. And, Houston, we do have a problem. All you have to do is traverse a mall and check out the packs of pudgy preadolescents waddling in your direction or read the umpteenth newspaper story about the childhood obesity "epidemic" plaguing our country. The hot topic is even the subject of a reality show. *Honey, We're Killing the Kids!*, broadcast on the TLC cable network, features clueless parents and chubby children receiving tough love from nutrition specialist Lisa Hark, Ph.D.

This is how TV reviewer Bill Gibron explained the premise of the hour-long program:

> Investing her angry schoolmarm shtick with good-natured gravitas, Dr. Hark is introduced to a family in need, then sets out to diagnose their failings. The entire brood is given a good going over from both medical and lifestyle standpoints. Tests are run, household habits are scrutinized. Using morphing techniques that resemble a beer-bellied version of Michael Jackson's "Black and White," Dr. Hark gives her charges the incredibly bad news: if Mom and Dad don't stop larding their offspring with crap, by age forty, the kids will look like broken down, alcoholic Teamsters."[1]

Go Figure

Although nearly two-thirds of Americans are overweight, 83 percent of us say our eating habits are very healthy or somewhat healthy, according to a Thomson Medstat survey. Only 3 percent of Americans characterized their eating habits as "not at all healthy."[2]

I've looked in on *Honey, We're Killing the Kids!*, and invariably, after Dr. Hark lays down the new rules, the roly-poly kids—whose dinners have revolved around chicken nuggets, boxed macaroni and cheese, and soggy microwave pizza—must suddenly eat "real" foods totally foreign to their taste buds, like fresh salads and steamed vegetables. What usually happens next on camera breaks my heart. The brats either throw a major hissy fit and refuse to eat their vegetables, or they nervously slip a forkful of broccoli into their mouths, only to throw it up on their plates.

Why do these kids upchuck healthy vegetables? The likely answer is that they've never been fed these nutritious foods before, which illustrates the loss of parental leadership, as I mentioned in the Introduction. In addition, I can point to several other reasons contributing to the societal mess we're in today:

- **Social changes.** The last half century has seen upheaval on the home front with the phenomenal rise of single-parent households and two-income families. These days many moms *have* to work because they're single parents or there's a pressing financial need to augment the family income. Other mothers work outside the home because they're more career minded. No matter what the reason, these sociological trends have impacted after-school routines and the way families eat dinner. Regarding the former, latchkey kids are told to stay inside the house because it's safe. There isn't much to do except veg out in front of the TV, play video games, and raid the cookie jar, which is filled with processed treats like Double Stuf Oreos or Keebler Chips Deluxe cookies.

  As for the way families eat dinner, in the past a stay-at-home mom's job description included the preparation of tasty, nutritious meals using fresh ingredients. These days, when bushed moms arrive home from work, they've got to get the laundry going, clean up around the house, tend to the children's homework, start the baths, *and* prepare dinner. The result: kids are raised on a rotation of delivery pizza, fast-food runs, microwave dinners, and Hamburger Helper–type meals.

  There's another aspect here worth mentioning. Since working parents have less time to shower their children with attention and playful activities, they reward them with "treats" like Pizza Hut dinners and Dairy Queen Blizzards as a way to assuage parental guilt. That's a shame because a better parental extravagance would be a home-cooked meal of organic chicken and whole grain pasta with a garden salad.

The Kids' Menu: Nothing but Junk

If your child can already read, he or she needn't bother perusing the kid's menu at a sit-down restaurant. I bet both of you can recite the children's menu by rote: chicken nuggets with fries, burger with fries, hot dog with fries, and macaroni and cheese, which may or may not come with fries.

I don't want to come across as a food snob, but I doubt the Rubin family will be frequenting the type of restaurant that serves breaded chicken fingers and fries for the kiddie crowd. When we go out to eat as a family, we gravitate toward restaurants that serve wild-caught tuna or sockeye salmon. Even chain restaurants, including Asian-fusion restaurants like P.F. Chang's, as well as good Thai restaurants, work well for us. It's also fun to order two or three main dishes and share them all.

Choose your restaurants carefully. Otherwise, you risk turning what should be an enjoyable family occasion—eating out—into a frustrating experience, especially if your children whine about not being able to order something off the kids' menu.

- **The rise of convenience foods.** Our supermarket aisles and refrigerator cases are filled with convenience foods that dispense with the hassle of preparing three square meals a day or after-school snacks. While food manufacturers have come up with ingenious ways to save time in the kitchen, store-bought meals are loaded with preservatives, processed ingredients, artificial flavors, synthetic colors, and trans fats. In more and more homes, it's not what's being peeled, chopped, or grilled any longer;

it's what's heating up in the microwave. Anytime your food has been produced by assembly-line workers in white lab coats and hairnets and radiated with ions, it won't be as healthy for you as fresh organic meats, vegetables, and fruits.

- **Fast food *über alles*.** You know the scenario: It's 6 p.m., and the last soccer practice is over. The kids are cranky with hunger, and you've got nothing in the refrigerator. The main boulevard is lined with every fast-food joint known to man, each one beckoning you to pull into its parking lot or drive-thru. Few hungry families can resist the siren call of cheesy chalupas, deep-dish pizza, mesquite bacon cheeseburgers, and "original recipe" fried chicken because their taste buds have been adulterated by the purveyors of fast food.

  Eric Schlosser, author of *Fast Food Nation*, says that millions of parents lead their children into fast-food restaurants every day without thinking through the ramifications. "They rarely consider where this food came from, how it was made, or what it is doing to the community around them," he wrote. Families just grab their plastic trays off the counter, find a table, unwrap their food, and dig in, unaware that they are participating in a transitory experience that's soon forgotten. "They should know what really lurks between those sesame-seed buns," said Schlosser. "As the old saying goes: You are what you eat."[3]

- **Advertising.** Food and beverage companies are spending $15 billion a year on television ads to entice children to eat massive amounts of unhealthy food, according to the Institute of Medicine.[4] If you plop your children in front of the TV on a Saturday morning, their sponge-like brains will soak in 130 food-related advertisements.[5] When Burger King had a commercial tie-in with *Teletubbies*, they sold chicken nuggets shaped like Tinky Winky, Dipsy, Laa-Laa, and Po. Even commercial-free PBS shows like *Sesame Street* allow Ronald McDonald and Chuck E. Cheese to drop by for a visit. Not so coincidentally, I might add.

The New Math

The third-grade teacher saw that little Johnny wasn't paying attention in class. "Johnny!" she called out from the blackboard. "What are 2 and 4 and 14 and 24?"

Little Johnny thought for a moment before the answer came to him: "NBC, FOX, ESPN, and the Cartoon Network!"

A Federal Communications Commission task force, made up of FCC officials; members of the food, television, and advertising industries; and various consumer health experts, began studying the link between viewing habits and childhood obesity in 2007. It will be interesting to read the final report. Since the FCC estimates that children watch between two and four hours of TV per day and view a barrage of forty thousand TV ads every year[6]—most of them for sugary cereal, chocolate candy, and fast food—I'm not sure what conclusion could be rendered except for the obvious: a barrage of junk food ads spurs junk food sales.

The reason junk food advertisers saturate the airwaves is because they're aware that children have "pester power," a unique way to nag their parents into buying something they want. These desires are created by catchy advertisements that rely on cute characters like SpongeBob SquarePants and good ol' Tony the Tiger to make the pitch for Kelloggs' Wild Bubble Berry Pop-Tarts or Kelloggs' Frosted Flakes, respectively. Young children, lacking discernment because of their immaturity, then repetitively whine ("Mom, Mom, Mom") while pleading their case ("All my friends love them!") until their parents acquiesce to their demands.

- **Movie tie-ins.** Just about any time a Pixar, DreamWorks, or Disney movie is released for the G-rated munchkin crowd, you can count on some type of promotional tie-in—from package labeling on candy wrappers to colorful Happy Meal boxes—featuring the animated film characters. The beloved Shrek character, which belongs to DreamWorks, appears in McDonald's ads. *Ice Age* merchandise is found in sugar-saturated cereals like Cocoa Krispies, Froot Loops, Honey Smacks, and Frosted Flakes. One back scratches the other.

"In an era when childhood obesity is exploding, it's a scandal that our entertainment elite has been blinded by the easy money they're getting from letting huggable movie characters pitch fat-saturated food," writes *Los Angeles Times* Calendar columnist Patrick Goldstein.[7] That's what is happening, although the Walt Disney Company has announced that it will be phasing out licensing deals with McDonald's in 2008 after declaring Buzz Lightyear and Lightning McQueen won't endorse junk food anymore. Cachow to that, but I'll believe it when I see it.

- **Sports celebrity endorsements.** Ever since slugger Babe Ruth was hired to endorse Red Rock Cola in the 1930s, companies have handsomely paid famous athletes to down their drinks or take a big bite of their food for the cameras. TV commercials and print ads are usually money well spent because consumers are more likely to buy products that have been endorsed by sports celebrities with high Q scores, the industry standard for measuring the appeal of a certain athlete. Michael Jordan and Yao Ming have pitched Big Macs for years. Ice princess Michelle Kwan attached her sweetheart image to Coca-Cola, while British soccer legend David Beckham bends it for Pepsi and Snickers candy bars.

    Some professional athletes unwittingly give free advertising. Golfer John Daly, known to put up low numbers on the golf course, boasts about the big numbers of Diet Cokes that he drinks every day. In his autobiography, Daly says he downs twenty Diet Cokes per day, or an astounding 7,120 cans a year, which makes for a lot of empties in that $1.3 million, forty-five-foot Featherlite Prevost motor home he travels around in.[8]

The Newest Extreme Sport

Just as today's toddlers are growing up in an era of extreme sports—skateboarding, snowboarding, and anything part of the X Games—they are being exposed to a new form of sporting entertainment: extreme eating. The cable sports network ESPN breathlessly covers Nathan's Famous International Hot Dog Eating Contest, held every summer at Coney Island, with all the hype of an NFL playoff game.

Since 2005, Paul Page has been ESPN's play-by-play announcer for the event, with Richard Shea as the color man. I can overhear them now:

Paul Page: *Look at the way Joey "Jaws" Chesnut is dunking his dogs in water to make them slide down his throat better.*

Richard Shea: *Joey better watch it. He doesn't want to vomit in this pressure situation, or he'll be DQ'd.*

In 2007, Joey Chesnut beat Takeru "Tsunami" Kobayashi, who won the Nathan's Famous International Hot Dog Eating Contest six years in a row and set all sorts of records in the nascent sport of "competitive eating." Joey gulped sixty-six hot dogs in twelve minutes, leaving Kobayashi in the dust and wondering if "Jaws" Chesnut should be tested for steroids.

Just kidding.

It Starts with You

Even though the popular culture is banging the drum loudly for junk foods, we—the parents—remain the strongest influence in our children's lives. Yes, I've heard that parental influence becomes more difficult when our offspring reach the challenging adolescent years, but this only underscores the importance of training them up in the way they should go while they are still young. Deuteronomy 11:19 reminds parents to teach principles of godly living and healthy behavior, 24/7: "You shall teach them to your children, speaking of them when you sit in your house, when you walk by the way, when you lie down, and when you rise up" (NKJV).

I believe that feeding children the most healthful foods *and* preparing fresh meals rank at the top among parental responsibilities, right below raising them in the "training and admonition of the Lord" (Eph. 6:4 NKJV). If you aren't nodding your head in agreement, it's my contention that your children aren't eating healthy foods because their *parents* aren't eating healthy foods.

What About You?

New research by Leanna L. Birth and colleagues at Penn State University found that fathers and mothers who had high calorie intakes—in other words, possessed a weakness for junk food—were raising children who weighed more than they should. The Penn State researchers concluded that a parent's poor choices in eating, along with little or no physical activity, were solid predictors of a child's risk of obesity.[9]

I can't tell you the number of mothers who, deeply concerned about how overweight and unhealthy their children are, seek me out after I speak in churches around the country. When these anxious moms approach me, fretfully working a tissue in their hands, I know what they're going to say: "Jordan, all my kids want to eat is junk. How can I get them to eat healthier food?"

Invariably, before I answer their question, I ask one of my own: "Ma'am, what do you eat?"

I'll see heads slump once again because these mothers consume the same junk they feed their kids. That doesn't stop them, however, from making excuses: "I don't have time to shop for fresh foods . . . I'm too tired at the end of a long day." For many, the tyranny of the urgent prevents them from preparing healthy meals.

So Where Are Those Twinkies Coming From?
by Dr. Fiona Blair

I know what Jordan's talking about because I must see some of these same mothers in my examination room. I remember the time this one mom brought her eight-year-old son in for a checkup. The poor kid weighed 150 pounds, and he was a third grader!

"Dr. Blair," said the mother, "you've got to do something about this child."

"*I've* got to do something about this child?" I asked. (Like his ballooned physique was *my* fault!)

"Yes, because I don't know what else to do. Look at him. He's so big."

"Yes, he's overweight, but what kind of foods does he eat?"

"He eats nothing but junk. His favorite food is Twinkies. He eats Twinkies all day long—"

I cut her off right there. "Does he have a job?" I queried.

"No," she replied with a look that said, *What kind of question is that?*

"Does he drive?"

"No."

"Then where's he getting the Twinkies from?"

Now, *that* question really hit home. She looked down and tugged at her purse. "I buy them for him," she whispered.

"Why are you doing that?"

She had no answer for me. Although it seemed simple and obvious to me that if you don't *buy* Twinkies, he won't *eat* Twinkies, that simple fact had eluded her.

I let this idea settle in before I offered some doctorly advice. "Now, let me remind you that you're in control of what he eats. It's not up to me to do something about it; it's up to *you*."

I practice what I preach. For instance, I leave a bowl of various fruits out for my children to snack on when they come home from school. I know that if I set a plate of doughnuts next to the fruit, the doughnuts will get eaten before the fruit, so I don't make the doughnut option available.

It's as simple as that.

This type of thinking is shortsighted because what you feed your kids today impacts their health . . . right now! The principles behind *The Great Physician's Rx for Children's Health*, which starts with Key #1, "Teach Them to Eat to Live," means following these two basic principles:

1. Serve foods that God created.
2. Serve foods in a form that is healthy for the body.

Servings foods that God created means shopping for foods as close to the natural source as possible. I'm talking about:

- whole grains, like wheat and barley;
- nuts and seeds;
- healthy dairy products, like yogurt, cheese, and butter;
- healthy red meats, like grass-fed beef, lamb, venison, and bison;
- cold-water fish caught in the wild; and, of course,
- a wide array of organically grown fruits and vegetables.

These nourishing foods will give your children the nutrients they need to build strong bones and young bodies, which is super important since they only grow to maturation once.

Let me illustrate some differences between foods that God created versus foods that man created. Today, many parents of toddler-age children have no problem feeding their bambinos Cheerios or Goldfish crackers as a quick snack.

Compared to lollipops or Tootsie Rolls, a handful of round O's from a box of General Mills Cheerios or crunchy Goldfish crackers from Pepperidge Farm are practically health foods in their minds.

Out of the Mouths of Babes

To the best of our knowledge, Joshua has eaten smiley Goldfish just one time. It happened in the church nursery when he was twenty-seven months old. On this occasion, my son grabbed a few Goldfish from another kid's plate.

When someone in the nursery told me what happened, I picked up my son and said, "Joshua, Goldfish are yucky," and pretty much left it at that.

A week later, I was packing up to leave the house, and I turned and announced in a chirpy voice, "Joshua, we're going to church tonight."

He looked at me and said, "Goldfish are yucky."

Joshua remembered.

A serving size of Cheerios (one cup, or about a fistful of the round oats cereal) has 110 calories and is touted on its distinctive canary-yellow box as low in fat and saturated fat, with no cholesterol. I think it would be instructive to take a closer look at Cheerios' ingredients, which I've listed here, followed by my commentary:

- **Whole grain oats.** All grains, when grown in the field, have three parts: bran, germ, and endosperm. Bran, the protective outer shell, is high in fiber and B vitamins. Germ, the seed for the new plant, contains B vitamins and some protein, minerals, and healthy oils. Endosperm contains starch, protein, vitamins, and minerals. Whole grain oats, as the main ingredient, sounds good for you, and there's no doubt that whole grain is better than "enriched" grains, which contain only the endosperm.

  The problem is that the phrase "whole grain oats" doesn't tell you very much about where the oats came from or if they're from 100 percent good sources. A supplier could even sprinkle whole grain oats into a mixture of enriched grains and legally call the ingredient "whole grain oats." The Whole Grains Council is trying to help consumers sort out the confusion by having manufacturers imprint black-and-gold stamps stating how many grams of whole grains you're receiving in a single serving size, but that standard has yet to be adopted across the board by the food industry.

At the end of the day, the fact that Cheerios' whole grain oats are not organically produced sends up a red flag in my book and most likely means they were grown on farmlands treated with toxic pesticides and fertilizers. In addition, these whole grains may have come from biotechnological crops that were genetically modified, meaning that scientists fiddled with the plant's genetic composition to boost crop yields. Genetically modified organisms (GMO) in grains have been the source of international controversy because of questions about their environmental safety.

Agricultural Asbestos?

You probably have no idea that you and your children have been eating genetically modified foods for some time. While you may not find many GMO whole fruits or vegetables in your local supermarket, an estimated 75 percent of the processed foods in this country (breakfast cereals, baked goods, vegetable oils, etc.) contain a potpourri of genetically modified organisms.[10] I find this to be an amazing development because GMO crops such as corn, soybeans, and potatoes have only been around since the mid-1990s.

Called the "food of the future" by proponents and "Frankenfood" by detractors, GMO crops are created by taking genes from one organism—often a mutated virus—and inserting them into another to make them grow higher, larger, denser, and more resistant to insect infestation. Those are all laudable goals, but the problem is that scientists are adding a gene to a food that wasn't originally part of that food, which is unnatural and changes the DNA character of the crop. I will not knowingly eat a product made from genetically modified ingredients because we don't know what their short-term or long-term effects might be.

I've been greatly influenced by Jeffrey Smith's book *Genetic Roulette*, which marshals the latest information on GMO foods. (He also quips that GMO should stand for "God Move Over.") I am more determined than ever to keep these dangerous genetically modified foods out of cupboards and refrigerators and off the kitchen tables of those I care about. Besides, why should I put myself, or my family, at risk when wonderful organic foods that God created are readily available for purchase?

- **Modified cornstarch.** It didn't take long for the Cheerios ingredients list to go downhill rapidly. Modified cornstarch is a thickening agent that has been "modified" through chemical reactions, but we're not told how it happened. A high percentage of modified cornstarch produced in the United States is genetically modified. In fact, if the labeling on the food product you're buying *doesn't* say GMO-free or non-GMO, you should assume that is contains GMOs.

- **Cornstarch.** This starch is used as another flavoring and thickening agent and has industrial uses as well in the manufacturing of adhesives and in laundry starch.

- **Sugar.** One serving size of Cheerios—30 grams—has one gram of sugar, which is one-fourth of a teaspoon. While Cheerios aren't known for being particularly sweet, I'm sure that General Mills adds sugar to the ingredients to make the cereal sweet enough to appeal to young palates. A quarter of a teaspoon may not sound like much, but when sugar is added to practically all processed foods, kids will notice when there *isn't* a sweet aftertaste—and they won't want to eat that food. I believe sugar, in its various forms, is the main reason we have a childhood obesity epidemic today. According to the *Journal of Pediatrics,* children get almost five hundred calories a day from candy, cookies, and snacks.

- **Salt.** A serving of Cheerios contains 250 milligrams of salt, which is 11 percent of the American Heart Association's recommendation of 2,300 milligrams of sodium daily. That's a lot for just one handful of cereal. The problem is that kids who eat boxed cereal or ham and eggs in the morning, turkey sandwiches and chips for lunch, and take-out pepperoni pizza and toasted garlic bread for dinner are probably taking in between 4,000 and 6,000 milligrams a day, making them prime candidates for high blood pressure when they become adults.

- **Tocopherols.** Time to pull out a medical dictionary. Tocopherols, which are antioxidants and a type of vitamin E, are found in corn, soybeans, and olive oil. They are no doubt used as a preservative to prevent food spoilage. What the label does not tell you is whether or not the tocopherols were produced artificially.

- **Trisodium phosphate.** This thickening agent known as TSP is widely available in hardware stores—where it's sold as a cleaning agent and degreaser.

- **Calcium carbonate.** Found naturally in minerals, rocks, and seashells, calcium carbonate is a source of dietary calcium.

- **Natural color.** I have no idea what "natural color" is, but it sounds better than artificial color. Still, it's likely made from a combination of questionable materials.

Now let's look at the other popular snack for the preschool set, cheddar cheese–flavored Pepperidge Farm Goldfish, which has the following ingredients:

- unbleached enriched wheat flour [flour, niacin, reduced iron, thiamin mononitrate (vitamin B1), riboflavin (vitamin B2), folic acid]

- cheddar cheese (pasteurized milk, cheese culture, salt, enzymes, water, salt)
- partially hydrogenated vegetable shortening (canola, soybean, cottonseed and/or sunflower oils)
- 2 percent or less of salt, yeast, sugar, and yeast extract
- leavening (baking soda, monocalcium phosphate)
- spices
- annatto (for color)
- onion powder

One ounce of Goldfish contains 140 calories, six grams of fat, and 230 milligrams of sodium, but more importantly, the snack is pretty much a zero in nutrients such as vitamins. Goldfish are high in iron, but that's it.

Compare these processed foods with what Nicki and I have been regularly packing in Joshua's backpack when he marches off to Sunday school or his morning preschool—flaxseed crackers. We like flaxseed crackers produced by a local farm, which has a rather simple list of ingredients on the box:

- organic flaxseeds
- organic vine ripened tomatoes
- organic green bell peppers
- organic red bell peppers
- organic orange bell peppers
- fresh organic cilantro
- organic scallions
- Celtic Sea Salt
- organic cayenne

Another flaxseed cracker we buy is Life Force Sun-Flax Originals, which contains raw organic sunflower seeds, raw organic flaxseeds, raw organic agave nectar, and Celtic Sea Salt.

So tell me: which snacks were made with foods that God created, and which snacks were a combination of genetically modified grains, thickening agents, and hydrogenated oils?

The answer is obvious, which illustrates a larger point: every chance you get, you should shop for items made with foods that God created, not something that man constructed. Eating organically exposes you and the children to foods that are far superior in taste and quality and reduces your exposure to chemicals and pesticides prevalent in conventionally produced food. Organic food is plain healthier for you and the family.

In fairness, I must point out that eating organically is not the whole answer since many unhealthy foods and ingredients—white flour, white sugar, pasteurized and homogenized dairy, and various vegetable oils—can come from organically grown sources, but they are not foods in the form that God created them.

The Newest Diversion: Extreme Eating

Eating junk food—like gambling—is a progressive addiction. That's the only way I can account for the growing popularity of some absolutely perverted eats. I'm talking about deep-fried Twinkies, deep-fried Oreos, deep-fried Snickers bars, and deep-fried Coke.

How do you deep-fry a *soft drink*? By soaking wet pancake batter with Coca-Cola and dropping it into a vat of boiling grease. Top the fried globs of Coke with a drizzle of chocolate syrup, a dusting of cinnamon sugar, and a dollop of whipped cream, and you have a real gut bomb.

You usually have to swing by street carnivals or state fairs to find delicacies like deep-fried peanut butter, jelly, and banana sandwiches or deep-fried macaroni-and-cheese, served on a stick, of course. At the Los Angeles

County Fair, vendor Charlie Boghosian is credited, if I may use that word, with inventing the Krispy Kreme Chicken and Swiss Sandwich, which is basically a chicken patty and a slice of gooey Swiss cheese slapped between slices of a Krispy Kreme doughnut.

Boghosian said he sold nearly one thousand of these sandwiches, at $5.95 a pop, the first weekend he unveiled them.[11]

Turning the Ship Around

Key #1, "Teach Them to Eat to Live" starts with you, the parent. You decide what you put into your shopping cart. You possess the power to decide everything your children eat inside the home. You set the example of what makes a delicious meal or nutritious snack.

The fact is that kids can't eat junk if there isn't any junk in the house. So does that mean I recommend setting a dumpster in the driveway and emptying your pantry and freezer of all the not-so-healthy foods? Not necessarily. You might have to quell a full-scale rebellion from youngsters who're addicted to Cocoa Puffs, Lay's Potato Chips, and Now and Later candies if you tossed out everything in a single afternoon. Because children are creatures of habit, the type who insist on a ham sandwich every day for lunch, it would be prudent to follow a more incremental approach, especially for older kids.

The small-step-at-a-time method is how I handled the food situation following my marriage to Nicki. I knew before she walked down the aisle that we weren't on the same page when it came to eating only foods that God created in a form healthy for the body. One thing I found out during our courtship was that I couldn't "force" Nicki, who was in her midtwenties and fairly set in her ways, to follow the Great Physician's prescription for health and wellness: I had to lead by example. To her credit, Nicki didn't have far to go. She didn't frequent McDonald's or drink Coke, but she did possess a weakness for Twizzlers and sweet tea by the gallon.

After settling into our apartment in West Palm Beach, we struck our first marital compromise: she would shop for her favorite foods at the local Publix supermarket, and I would pick up grass-fed beef, free-range chicken, frozen foods, salads, fruits, and snacks—all organic—at Nutrition World, a local health food store.

One night, I brought home an Amy's 3 Cheese Pizza—not the world's healthiest food, but still a totally organic and utterly great-tasting pizza. (Neither of us cooked much in the early days of our marriage.) After heating my pizza alongside her store-bought version in the oven, I offered Nicki a slice of Amy's 3 Cheese Pizza. Her taste buds burst with appreciation. "That tastes good! Way better than mine," she agreed. Another time, for dessert, I asked Nicki if she wanted to sample one of my Pamela's Peanut Butter cookies, which were wheat-free organic treats. She found them scrumptious and nearly finished the box.

Over the next month or two, Nicki slowly but surely made the switch: whatever I ate, she ate as well. Then she overcame her lack of aptitude for cooking when she discovered that she was quite capable of cooking fresh fish or free-range chicken in a saucepan with some organic vegetables. Dicing up some garlic and cooking everything in organic butter could make anything taste good. Today, Nicki is a marvelous cook who could hang with the celebrity chefs on the Food Network. She loves to experiment with recipes like spinach-and-goat-cheese lasagna, made with ground buffalo meat.

When it comes to your family, I would suggest making subtle but strategic changes in what you serve them. In a nutshell, I'm talking about:

- less fast food and more home-cooked meals;

- fewer processed meals-in-a-box and more free-range chicken breasts, diced up and sautéed in butter, onions, and garlic;

- fewer canned vegetables and fruit in syrup and more organic vegetables and fruits fresh from the fields; and

- fewer sugary treats and more snack-time discipline.

The children must see you *and* your spouse eating healthfully, or they won't buy into the new program. As for how quickly you want to make the transition, you're welcome to attempt a total health makeover if you feel your sons and daughters are ready for that, but many children need time to be retrained in the way they should go.

Joseph Mercola, an osteopathic physician and founder of the influential health Web site www.mercola.com, reminds parents that training your children to eat the right foods is a marathon, not a sprint. "If you start to do some food Nazi, dictatorial type of recommendations, this will be absolutely counter-productive . . .The goal of training your children is to help them learn exactly what they are designed to eat so that they can choose foods that will keep them healthy for the rest of their lives, but if you take a rigid approach, you run the risk of having them rebel on you once they get out of your supervision."[12]

To help you see how "Eat to Live" works, I've come up with Ten Command-ments that you would be wise to follow. Here they are:

I. THOU SHALT SHOP FOR ORGANIC WHOLE FOODS

Ninety percent of Americans' household food budget is spent on processed foods, the majority of which are filled with additives and stripped of nutrients.[13]

This will have to change.

The Great Physician's prescription begins with you making a conscious decision to shop for organic whole foods. I'm referring to fruits, vegetables, and grains that haven't been doused with chemical pesticides, herbicides, and synthetic fertilizers; dairy products and meats coming from livestock that chew fresh grass in open fields or on organic feed that hasn't been laced with antibiotics and growth hormones; and prepackaged and ready-to-eat foods produced from organic ingredients, like Joshua's flaxseed crackers.

Eating organically grown foods not only reduces the intake of toxins into young bodies, but they also pack more nutritional punch. This is an important distinction because the nutrient content of conventionally grown fruits and vegetables has dropped markedly since the 1950s, according to a University of

Texas study headed by biochemist Donald R. Davis, Ph.D. After studying historic and current US Department of Agricultural data on forty-three garden crops, such as vegetables, strawberries, and melons, Dr. Davis discovered that modern produce has lost protein (down an average of 6 percent), calcium (down 16 percent), vitamin C (down 20 percent), riboflavin (down 38 percent), and phosphorus (down 9 percent).[14] Another study showed that organically grown strawberries contain 19 percent more antioxidants, which prevent cell damage, than conventionally grown strawberries.

For decades, we've been sacrificing food quality for quantity by devising methods to hike crop yields through chemical fertilization, pesticide use, and genetic engineering. That model is being turned upside down as millions of families learn about the health hazards of conventionally grown foods, discover how wonderful organic whole foods taste, and experience how much "cleaner" they feel.

A decade ago, organic food sales represented less than 1 percent of total food and beverage sales, but that figure has climbed to 2.5 percent and continues to maintain rapid growth of 20 percent a year, an incredible development.[15] To meet this increasing demand, natural food markets like Whole Foods, Wild Oats, and Sprouts are opening by the droves in downtown storefronts and suburban malls. Traditional grocers like Kroger, Publix, and Safeway are responding to this growing market by stocking organic fruits, vegetables, and dairy products.

If you want to look to the future for organic food shopping, look no farther than San Diego, where I lived back in 1996 at the age of twenty-one during my comeback from terrible illnesses that struck me while I was a Florida State University student. While recuperating in America's Finest City, I was committed to eating as organically as possible, but I was limited to shopping at Boney's, a chain of natural grocery stores in the San Diego area, and places like the Ocean Beach People's Organic Food Co-op. These were the only markets where I could purchase wild-caught salmon, pesticide-free lettuce and tomatoes, certified raw kefir and cream, and raw cheeses.

How things have changed in a decade! On a recent visit to San Diego, I learned there are now more than *thirty dozen* natural food stores in the county, including Whole Foods, Trader Joe's, Jimbo's, Windmill Farms, Sprouts, Bristol Farms, and Henry's Farmers Markets (formerly Boney's and now corporately owned by Wild Oats). These stores offer a colorful variety of foods that God created in a form healthy for the body. Another personal favorite is Trader Joe's, found mainly on the west and east coasts—but not in Florida yet. Trader Joe's is a must-stop for me whenever I'm in New York or California.

And then there is Wal-Mart. In 2006, the world's largest retailer and number-one seller of groceries began offering a thousand organic products at a target price of just 10 percent more than conventional food, which made organic food more affordable overnight. Wal-Mart is the eight-hundred-pound gorilla that has the potential—through its tremendous purchasing power—to send ripples through the global economy. For instance, in just a year or two, Wal-Mart became the world's biggest seller of organic milk. By creating more consumer demand for organic foods, farmers and ranchers will have the financial incentive to switch over to raising organic crops, dairy, and livestock.

"What Wal-Mart has done is legitimized the market [for organic food]," said Harvey Hartman, president of a consulting group working with Wal-Mart on its organic food initiatives. "All these companies who thought organics was a niche product now realize that it has an opportunity to become a big business."[16]

Major grocery chains have noticed the shift in customer attitudes toward organics and are not sitting idly by. Albertsons, Ralphs, Fred Meyer, Kroger, Winn-Dixie, Safeway, Vons, and even our excellent local grocery store, Publix, are dedicating entire aisles to organic foods and revamping their fruit and produce sections with hardwood floors, soft lighting, and earth-toned color schemes. Warehouse clubs like Sam's Club (owned by Wal-Mart) and Costco are jumping in as well, selling organic eggs, wild-caught fish, and organic frozen berries, perfect for breakfast smoothies.

You have other options besides Wal-Mart, Whole Foods, or supermarkets. Farmer's markets are great places to find locally grown fruits and vegetables raised without pesticides and herbicides, but they are often set up only one day a week in a town square. Buying local is great for your children's health and for the environment. Roadside stands are another source for local foods, but they are usually open just during the season.

Don't Forget Health Food Stores!

Although I can appreciate the jazzy environment of a Whole Foods or the eclectic mix of tantalizing foods at Trader Joe's, I still have a soft spot in my heart for the mom-and-pop health food stores that have been the backbone of the organic movement for decades. Long before Whole Foods came to Palm Beach Gardens, I shopped at Nutrition World, an independent health food store where I worked as a stock boy when I was ten years old. I also patronize Nutrition S'Mart because I like their organic products and their service.

Your local independent health food store—check it out.

II. THOU SHALT READ FOOD PACKAGING AND NUTRITION FACTS

Just as you can't tell who the players are without a program, you won't have an idea of what you're buying until you understand the terminology on the product packaging. Food producers must meet standards set by the US Department of Agriculture before a food can be labeled as "organic." In a nutshell, organic produce cannot be grown with pesticides or most synthetic fertilizers, and animals cannot be injected with antibiotics and growth hormones. Organic farms undergo a rigorous certification process and are inspected for compliance by an independent agent.

Here's what the following descriptions mean:

- **100% Organic.** The food must be all-organic or contain only organically produced ingredients.
- **Organic.** The food must be at least 95 percent organic.

- **Made with Organic Ingredients.** The food must contain at least 70 percent organic ingredients.

- **All Natural.** Meaningless, I'm afraid. No standard definition exists except when it's applied to meat and poultry products; otherwise, the food manufacturer alone decides whether to use it. Case in point: 7Up, the soft drink, advertises itself as "100 percent natural," claiming with a straight face that one of its five ingredients—high fructose corn syrup— is a natural ingredient.

Another shopping must is reading the "Nutrition Facts" found on every food item for sale in America. I will not drop anything in my shopping cart— even if I'm shopping at Whole Foods, Trader Joe's, or Joe Bob's Natural Food Emporium—without reading what ingredients are in the food. I scan the labels for buzzwords like enriched flour, partially hydrogenated oils, color dye, and unpronounceable names for chemical preservatives. I look for sugar masquerading behind names like corn syrup, high fructose syrup, sucrose, sorbitol, dextrose, glucose, corn sweetener, sorghum syrup, and fruit juice concentrate. While traveling through Switzerland a couple of years ago, Nicki and I shopped for picnic lunches in supermarkets, and by Swiss law the manufacturer must print the ingredients in three languages—German, French, and Italian—on their food labels. I learned quickly that *zucker*, *sucre*, and *zucchero* meant the same thing in English: sugar.

Studying food labels, however, doesn't guarantee that you're buying the healthiest food. Deceptive labeling, unfortunately, is rampant in the food industry. For instance, some manufacturers hide the presence of monosodium glutamate, a dangerous food additive also known as MSG, by listing the substance as autolyzed yeast extract. Some say the listings for calories, fat grams, sodium, and sugar reminds them of the Environmental Protection Agency's bogus estimates for gas mileage ratings on new cars.

Anytime I see the word *hydrogenated* next to "oil," I set the product back on the shelf because partially hydrogenated, fractionated, or hydrogenated oils contain trans fats, which have been called a "slow form of poison" by heart specialists.[17] Trans fats are killers: research shows that trans fats are twice as dangerous for your heart as saturated fat and the most detrimental contributor to cardiovascular health. A Harvard University nutrition expert, Walter C. Willet, M.D., called trans fats "the biggest food-processing disaster in US history,"[18] which explains why several major cities, such as New York City and Chicago, have passed laws banning restaurants from serving foods cooked with trans fats. Big Apple eateries must comply by July 1, 2008, which will be interesting to watch.

It's also been exciting to keep an eye on gigantic food conglomerates like Kraft and Nabisco. They've been falling over themselves to eliminate trans fats from their frozen pizzas, dip chips, and party crackers after food producers were ordered to list the number of trans fats in their foods in 2006. I'm pleased that the light of truth is forcing some corporate responsibility, but caveat emptor: laws are made to be broken, and there are always loopholes. Even though Nabisco rejiggered Oreos with zero fat grams, the popular sandwich cookie is still extremely unhealthy.

Do You Read Labels?

Nearly 80 percent of Americans insist that they read nutritional labels before they set the food item in their shopping carts, according to an Associated Press-Ipsos poll,[19] but that number sounds high to me, especially when you know that two-thirds of American adults weigh too much in this country. My thinking is that respondents would be too embarrassed to tell pollsters that they don't bother reading food labels, just as they fudge the truth about how often they go to church or vote.

My mother, who has been eating natural and organic foods for thirty-five years, is still fooled by bread that has "made with whole grains" on the label. Believe it or not, even the ingredient listed as "wheat flour" is actually white or unbleached wheat flour, not whole grain.

There's another "gotcha" in this food label game, and it's called *serving size.* Manufacturers will make their serving size as small as possible to fool you. Here's a common example: a 20-ounce Pepsi has a label stating that there are just 100 calories and 27 grams of sugar "per serving." It's not until you read the fine print that you discover a "serving size" is 8 ounces, meaning there are *two and a half* servings in that bottle of soda pop. That's ridiculous since no one buys a Pepsi with the intention of not drinking the entire bottle. Most consumers, who are in a hurry anyway, might glance at the nutritional label and think to themselves, *This Pepsi only has a hundred calories,* when in fact, they'd be guzzling 250 calories and 81 grams of sugar after finishing the last sip.

But you shouldn't be drinking Pepsi anyway. Nor should you be falling for the latest marketing craze—100-calorie snack packs. Nabisco doles out one hundred calories' worth of Oreos, Chips Ahoy, Cheese Nips, Wheat Thins, and Planters Peanut Butter Cookie Crisps in diminutive, individual portion packaging. So does Pringles.

It's a silly gimmick—and an expensive one at that. Don't let the junk food companies fatten up their bottom lines at the expense of your children's health.

Hey, Isn't Guacamole Supposed to Have Avocados?

You would think that peanut butter is made from peanuts, eggnog is made from eggs, and guacamole is made from avocados.

Not in the Alice in Wonderland world we live in, where "guacamole" dip has either no or almost no avocado but plenty of modified food starches, partially hydrogenated soybean and coconut oils, corn syrup, whey, and artificial colors like yellow #5 and blue #1 to give their dip that "avocadoey" look.

A Los Angeles women, Brenda Lifsey—like Claude Rains in the movie classic, *Casablanca*—was shocked, just shocked, to learn that a processed-foods giant like Kraft Foods would produce and sell a guacamole dip that contained less than 2 percent avocados. She filed a class-action lawsuit in 2006 to stop Kraft from marketing the dip as guacamole. She also sought unspecified punitive damages.[20]

And Americans say they read food labels. Actually, this is proof that food conglomerates can put just about anything in a plastic tub and people will buy it, no questions asked!

III. Thou Shalt Feed Your Children Grass-Fed Beef, Pasture-Raised Chicken, and Wild-Caught Fish

Remember how I told you that my 70s-era parents—who were not quite hippies but were certainly countercultural—raised me as a granola kid? They also raised me as a vegetarian for the first four years of my life, which stopped when Mom became pregnant with my sister, Jenna. Mom felt she needed the nutrients only found in meat to nourish the life growing inside her, so she and Dad made the decision to reintroduce meat to the family dinner table. I remember that my Grandma Rose had the honor of handing me my first chicken leg.

I'm glad I gnawed on that roast chicken because my growing body needed the key essential amino acids found only in animal protein. This may surprise you, but I'm not in favor of vegetarianism or veganism, especially for small children who are years away from physical maturation. Feeding babies a vegan diet is particularly dangerous; in 2007, the parents of a six-week-old child, Crown Shakur, were convicted of murder, involuntary manslaughter, and cruelty for feeding their infant son a diet of soymilk and apple juice, which led to his death by starvation. This was at least the third such conviction of vegan parents since 2003.[21]

Vegetarianism, a relaxed form of veganism, has certainly caught on with the trendy celebrity set, many who view their decision not to "eat animals" as a cause célèbre. Hollywood actors Alec Baldwin, Danny DeVito, Dustin Hoffman, and comedian Jerry Seinfeld are reportedly vegetarians. Ex-Beatle Paul McCartney won't allow any meat or meat by-products in the backstage area while on tour.

Pamela Anderson of *Baywatch* fame says that when she drives by KFC, her kids ask her to honk, and they yell, "Boo" out the car window.[22]

The problem with vegetarian and vegan activism is human physiology. As my friend Sally Fallon, president of the Weston A. Price Foundation, points out in her book *Nourishing Traditions*, the health of the brain and nervous system are dependent upon receiving certain amino acids—methionine, cysteine, and cystine—that are found plentifully in eggs and meat. Animal protein is our only source of complete protein, while protein sources from the vegetable kingdom contain only incomplete protein.

"Not only is it difficult to obtain adequate protein on a diet devoid of animal products, but such a diet often leads to deficiencies in many important minerals as well," wrote Sally Fallon. "This is because a largely vegetarian diet lacks the fat-soluble catalysts needed for mineral absorption . . . zinc, iron, calcium, and other minerals from animal sources that are easily and readily absorbed. We should not underestimate the dangers of deficiencies in these minerals," she said, adding that strict vegetarianism is particularly dangerous for growing children.[23]

Vegetarianism, while fashionable, is not widely embraced. In fact, you could say that Americans love their meat, eating it 4.2 times a week or 218 times a year,[24] and I'm confident that meat is a dinner-time staple in your home. There are considerable nutritional differences, however, between conventionally raised beef, production-line chicken, and farm-raised fish versus grass-fed beef, free-range chicken, and wild-caught fish.

My biggest problem with commercial meat is that cattle, chicken, and fish are raised and fattened on feed containing hormones, nitrates, and pesticides. Raising livestock on these types of grain is the equivalent of raising children on candy. Livestock and chickens are also penned up in conditions on "factory farms," which are also known as confined livestock operations (CLOs) or intensive livestock operations (ILOs). These factory farms confine hundreds to thousands of animals in impossibly cramped conditions with no access to sunlight, fresh air, or natural movement. According to the Grace Factory Farm Project, an estimated 70 percent of all antibiotics in the United States are fed to cattle, poultry, and pigs to promote growth and compensate for the unsanitary and deplorable living conditions on factory farms.[25] (To learn more about the untold story of conventional agriculture and factory farming, visit www.themeatrix.com and watch several of their clever animated features.)

The much healthier alternative is grass-fed beef produced from cattle that leisurely chew the cud on pastured grasslands, or free-range chickens that hunt and peck for their food in the outdoors. You and your children will be so much better off when you consume these organically raised meats, which are naturally leaner and contain larger concentrations of nutrients and healthy fats.

Wild-caught fish harvested by fishermen and fishing fleets in oceans and rivers are nutritionally better than "feedlot salmon," who pass their days making tight circles in long concrete sloughs and gulping food pellets. Fish caught in the wild are a richer source of omega-3 fats, key amino acids, potassium, vitamins, and minerals than farm-raised fish as well. You can purchase fresh, frozen, or canned wild Alaskan salmon and other wild-caught fish from your local fish market or health food store. Many other fish are healthy as well, including sardines, herring, mackerel, tuna, snapper, bass, and cod.

Choose "Sustainable" Wild Fish

Scientists at Dalhousie University in Halifax, Nova Scotia, are worried that stocks of commercial fishing species will collapse by 2048 due to overfishing. They say that 90 percent of the big fish—tuna, cod, and swordfish—are gone from the oceans and that only 6 percent of the global fish catch can be certified as "sustainable," meaning that fish are not pulled from the ocean any faster than they can reproduce.[26]

Colossal businesses like Wal-Mart, McDonald's, and Red Lobster restaurants are pressuring their suppliers to sell them only fish that meet international standards for sustainability. You can do your part for the environment—and help ensure that there will be a nutritious protein source for your children and children's children—by looking for the blue-and-white label from the Marine Stewardship Council that the fish are certified as sustainably caught.

I'm also a huge fan of lamb, known as an excellent source of zinc, a mineral critical to immune function as well as the healing of wounds like scraped knees from the playground. Lamb is high in vitamin B_{12}, which supports the production of red blood cells and allows nerve cells to develop properly, and carnitine, a nutrient important for a healthy heart. According to Sally Fallon, B_{12} deficiencies bring about pernicious anemia, impaired eyesight, panic attacks, schizophrenia, nervous disorders, and loss of balance.[27]

Americans eat a fraction of the amount of lamb consumed elsewhere in the world, which is a shame because this delicious red meat has a tender, buttery quality. We've become big lamb eaters in the Rubin household, and we all love lamb chops, rack of lamb, lamb burgers, lamb sausage, lamb in meat loaf, and barbecued lamb steaks. In fact, if you ask Joshua what his favorite foods are, don't be surprised if he mentions lamb.

IV. THOU SHALT EAT CULTURED, FERMENTED DAIRY PRODUCTS

One of the first things moms do so the family can "eat healthy" is purchase 2 percent or skim milk in place of whole milk. They've heard dieticians blame the saturated fats in whole milk for the spectacular rise in child obesity and heeded their counsel to shop for reduced-fat or fat-free skim milk.

The milk with blue or yellow caps has to be better for you than the red-cap stuff, right?

I could quip that I've never heard of a milking cow producing 2 percent or skim milk, but the reality is that removing the fat makes the milk less nutritious and less digestible, and can cause allergies. Furthermore, the homogenization of milk alters the fats and makes them more likely to damage arteries and potentially harm the body. For these reasons, I don't recommend children drinking *any* commercially pasteurized, homogenized milk, even if it is organic.

I realize that an explanation is called for. Up until the start of the twentieth century, people drank milk straight from the teats of cows and goats. "Sure, it was contaminated, but so was everything else," wrote William Campbell Douglass II, M.D. and author of *The Milk Book: The Milk of Human Kindness Is*

Not Pasteurized.[28] When cow's milk was bottled for sale and consumption, globules of butterfat separated from the milk and floated to the top of the bottle, which is where we received the expression: "The cream always rises to the top."

Milk producers thought that milk with the cream separated was unappetizing for consumers. Auguste Gaulin, a Frenchman, patented a nifty machine in 1899 that shot milk through a fine nozzle to break up the fat globules so that the butterfat would not rise to the top. This process became known as *homogenization*, but it didn't become popular until the 1930s.

What Have They Done to Milk?

America's favorite curmudgeon, Andy Rooney of *60 Minutes*, nailed it when he wondered during one of his Sunday night commentaries why people are drinking less milk than they used to. "Has it ever occurred to them that people aren't drinking it because milk isn't as good as it used to be?" he wondered.

"I like half and half on my shredded wheat but when I say 'half and half,' I mean half milk and half cream," Rooney explained. "I bought some half and half the other day and I didn't like the taste so I looked at the label . . . Listen to these ingredients: 'Nonfat milk, milk, corn syrup solids, artificial color, sugar, dipotassium phosphate, sodium citrate mono, and diglycerides, carrageenan, natural and artificial flavors, [and] vitamin A palmitate.' This is half and half? It's not half anything I want and it has nothing to do with something as good as milk."

Andy Rooney's suggestion to milk producers: "If they want to sell more milk . . . go back to selling what comes out of a cow."[29]

My thoughts precisely.

What researchers have learned is that the homogenization process creates an enzyme called *xanthine oxidase*, or "XO," which contributes to heart disease by damaging the arteries and building up arterial plaque. The milk industry says that pasteurization kills XO, which is highly debatable, but pasteurization also alters vital amino acids, which reduces a child's ability to access the proteins, fats, vitamins, and minerals in milk.

Heating the milk during pasteurization turns the milk sugar lactose into beta-lactose, which is more rapidly absorbed into the bloodstream and raises blood sugar levels. "The sudden rise in blood sugar is followed by a fall leading to low blood sugar, hypoglycemia, which induces hunger," wrote Dr. Douglass. "The end result is obesity. Obesity has become one of the most common diseases of childhood. Pasteurized milk makes you fat; raw milk does not."[30]

I've been heavily influenced by Dr. Douglass's *The Milk Book*, which makes a strong case for drinking certified or safe raw milk instead of the pasteurized, homogenized milk that fills the refrigerated cases of supermarkets. Unfortunately, certified raw milk is not widely available, thanks to the "Got Milk?" lobby and the National Dairy Council. I can't buy raw milk in Florida because it's illegal. A health food store near my home sells raw cow's and goat's milk, but there's a label slapped on the bottle stating, "For pet consumption only."

During my health recovery in the mid-1990s, I wanted to drink raw milk after reading the Bible—there was no pasteurization in the land of milk and honey—and Dr. Douglass's book. Since raw milk wasn't commercially available in Florida, I was forced to be creative. A good friend, Joanne Nightingale, owned a goat herd close to home. She helped nurse me back to health by giving me raw goat's milk and not accepting payment.

When Nicki started breast-feeding our son, she began having problems with engorgement, blocked ducts, and mastitis when Joshua was two or three months old. Her body couldn't produce enough milk for our hungry boy. We knew the last thing we wanted to feed Joshua was pasteurized cow's milk or commercial formula for reasons I've already mentioned. Necessity being the mother of invention, I devised an infant formula, based on suggestions from *Nourishing Traditions,* that would closely match the high-quality nutrients found in breast milk, though nothing can replace God's perfect design for breastfeeding.

Joshua's Formula

This is the infant formula I made after it became apparent that Nicki could no longer breastfeed our son. The formula can be used for infants up to eighteen months of age, the toddler formula for children up to three years of age. You can find suppliers and addresses for the ingredients by visiting www.BiblicalHealthInstitute.com and clicking on the Children's Formula icon.

I've shared these formulas with many friends who've used them with great success. But before using any infant or toddler formula, please consult with your pediatrician or family practitioner. No parents should use this information or start a nutritional program for their children without first seeking a doctor's advice.

Ingredients for Infant Formula (makes 38 ounces)

- 24 oz. spring water
- 12 oz. goat's milk (raw or pasteurized)
- 1/2 teaspoon children's probiotic powder
- 1/2 teaspoon acerola cherry powder (17 percent vitamin C)
- 2 teaspoons whey protein concentrate
- 2 teaspoons nutritional yeast
- 3 capsules buffalo liver or 3 capsules of colostrum
- 8 tablespoons mineral whey powder
- 1 teaspoon cod liver oil
- 1 teaspoon of butter oil
- 1 teaspoon sunflower oil
- 1 teaspoon extra virgin olive oil
- 2 teaspoons extra virgin coconut oil

Toddler Formula (makes 50 ounces)

- 32 oz. coconut water (from fresh young or Thai coconuts available at your local health food store)
- 16 oz. raw or pasteurized goat's milk, raw or pasteurized non-homogenized grass-fed cow's milk, or raw cow's milk colostrum
- $1/2$ teaspoon children's probiotic powder
- 1 teaspoon cod liver oil
- 1 teaspoon of butter oil or 1 teaspoon organic ghee (clarified butter)
- 1 teaspoon sunflower oil
- 1 teaspoon extra virgin olive oil
- 2 teaspoons extra virgin coconut oil

The major ingredient, I decided, would be raw goat's milk because it's an easily digestible protein that does not contain the same complex proteins found in cow's milk. Goat's milk has higher amounts of medium-chain fatty acids (MCFAs) than other milk and 7 percent less lactose than cow's milk. Furthermore, raw or cultured goat's milk fully digests in a baby's stomach in twenty minutes, while pasteurized cow's milk takes eight hours because of the difference in the goat milk's structure: its fats and protein molecules are tiny in size, which is the key to rapid absorption in the digestive tract.

I didn't have the time nor the inclination to meet a farmer in a back alley, so to speak, for a clandestine raw milk transaction. I had befriended Mark McAfee, owner of Organic Pastures Dairy (www.organicpastures.com) in Fresno, California, and he said he would be glad to ship me frozen raw cow's milk colostrum via UPS Next Day Air. (Raw milk can be legally sold in California and by mail order, as long as it's frozen.) Then I found another great source: Hendricks Farm & Dairy (www.hendricksfarmsanddairy.com) in Teleford, Pennsylvania, which is state licensed to sell raw milk.

Joshua has been consuming clean raw milk—mostly goat's milk, sheep's milk, and cow's milk colostrum—since we introduced him to the formula at three months of age and began giving it to him exclusively at six months. Nicki and I added yogurt to his diet when he celebrated his first birthday, and he absolutely loves sheep's milk yogurt. We serve him Old Chatham Sheepherding sheep's milk yogurt nearly every day. Sheep's milk dairy is more nutritious than either cow or goat's milk and is my personal favorite.

Got Raw Milk?

There are risks associated with consuming raw milk, so I only recommend purchasing raw milk from a certified or state-licensed source unless you are absolutely sure of the quality. Otherwise, you should use pasteurized, nonhomogenized milk in the homemade infant and toddler formulas. For more information on raw milk, visit www.realmilk.com.

Cultured dairy is an excellent source of easily digestible protein, B vitamins, probiotics, and calcium, the latter nutrient deemed vital to growing strong bones in children. Cultured dairy attacks bacterial infections, soothes the stomach lining, and prevents dental cavities.

For your children, I especially recommend raw goat and sheep cheese, which can be added to dinnertime salads, and yogurt made from sheep or goat's milk. Yes, there's a certain pungency to goat dairy products, but I find sheep's milk dairy to be creamy and delicious. I bet your toddler would love sheep or goat cheese in salad or on toast.

If you decide to buy commercial milk, make sure that you consume pasteurized but nonhomogenized milk, which is usually sold in glass bottles at the health food store. Goat's milk is another option because it is naturally homogenized and does not contain XO.

Do You Have a Lactose-Intolerant Child?
by Dr. Fiona Blair

I have many stressed-out mothers in my practice who are convinced that their children are intolerant to cow's milk–based formulas. I explain that children are rarely born lactose intolerant and most likely their son or daughter has an allergy to processed, pasteurized cow's milk. I usually try to get the mother to breast-feed exclusively and not supplement with a commercial formula, which usually fixes the problem, because human breast milk is the perfect food for infants.

However, if breast milk was never started, I often recommend a soy-milk formula because it's not a cow-based milk. There can be a problem with that since 30 percent of children are also allergic to soymilk, and soymilk presents its own challenges. (Visit www.westonaprice.org to learn about the potential dangers of soy-based formulas.) In these cases, we have to resort to elemental formulas on the market.

I also tell the parent that when the child is older and weaned off the breast, I recommend trying goat's milk before trying cow's milk again. Children manifest an allergy to cow's milk formula by gastrointestinal symptoms through vomiting and diarrhea; respiratory symptoms like constant sneezing, coughing, and congestion; and even with skin complications, like eczema. Those who are highly allergic need to use goat's milk or an elemental formula, like Jordan's homemade formula.

My response is that nearly all infants drink breast milk—their tender stomachs can't handle any solid foods—but breast milk has lactose. So breast milk, a food that God created to nourish and sustain newborns and infants while carrying the mother's antibodies to the baby, is obviously a good thing.

When infants are weaned from breast milk, they are fed formula—a highly processed dried dairy product made from cows that are not fed well or raised properly. Babies sometimes react poorly to commercial formula by screaming to the high heavens, prompting concerned mothers to immediately blame "lactose intolerance" as the cause of their child's ills.

Many switch to soymilk or a soy-based formula, but I'm no fan of soy products. Most soy protein comes from genetically modified soybeans. According to Sally Fallon, author of *Nourishing Traditions*, soybeans are high in phytic acid, which can block the complete intake of essential minerals like calcium, magnesium, copper, iron, and zinc into the intestinal tract. Soy protein must be processed at high temperatures to reduce phytic acid levels, which pretty much destroys the "good proteins" in soy, such as lysine.

Ms. Fallon points to research showing that soy formulas lack cholesterol (essential for brain development) and lactose and galactose, which play an equally important role in the development of the nervous system.

Most children are not lactose intolerant; otherwise, they couldn't tolerate breast milk. The reason for their stomach distress has more to do with an allergy or sensitivity to the processed protein in the formula, not any abdominal intolerance to lactose. If your child does not respond well to conventional infant formulas, look for a natural and organic infant formula at your local health food store or try the formula that I made for Joshua. I share the ingredients for that formula on pages 35–36.

V. THOU SHALT NOT EAT PORK OR SHELLFISH

You probably think I'm jumping from the frying pan into the fire with this commandment, but I mean it. I realize I'm talking about abstaining from some of America's favorite foods: hot dogs, bacon, pork chops, and barbecue, as well as shrimp, crab, and lobster.

Take the venerable hot dog. Please.

I realize that kids love eating hot dogs, and you may serve 'em so often that your children think they're one of the four major food groups. But hot dogs are vile meats, and the cliché is that you'd never eat one if you saw how they're made. The ingredients label may say that the hot dogs are made from "pork products," but the gut-wrenching reality is that hot dog manufacturers mix skeletal muscles with parts of pig's stomach, intestines, spleens, and leftover snouts and lips—yuck—in an industrial-sized blender, and, voilà, out come frankfurters/wieners/red hots ready for the next barbecue. During hot dog season—Memorial Day to Labor Day—Americans consume seven billion hot dogs, according to the National Hot Dog Council. Hot dogs carry a cancer risk for kids, as well: according to a research study of Los Angeles children ages ten and younger, children eating three hot dogs a week have nearly ten times the risk of leukemia as children who ate none.[31]

Another reason I'm down on this ballpark staple, an all-American food linked in the national conscious with Chevrolet and apple pie, is because God called pork a "detestable" and "unclean" meat in Leviticus 11 and Deuteronomy 14. It's right there in black and white, in God's own words:

> "You shall not eat any detestable thing. These are the animals which you may eat: the ox, the sheep, the goat, the deer, the gazelle, the roe deer, the wild goat, the mountain goat, the antelope, and the mountain sheep. And you may eat every animal with cloven hooves, having the hoof split into two parts, and that chews the cud, among the animals. Nevertheless, of those that chew the cud or have cloven hooves, you shall not eat, such as these: the camel, the hare, and the rock hyrax; for they chew the cud but do not have cloven hooves; they are unclean for you. Also the swine is unclean for you, because it has cloven hooves, yet does not chew the cud; you shall not eat their flesh or touch their dead carcasses." (Deut. 14:3–8 NKJV)

Question: Why did God inform the Israelites that they were not to eat pork? Was it because they couldn't lug refrigerators with them while they trekked forty years in the wilderness? No, God forbade pork because of the animal's physiology. Pigs have a simple stomach arrangement that takes the food in and rapidly passes it out the back end, which means that there's not enough time for the pig's simple digestive system to properly digest the food's nutrients or eliminate any wastes and toxins in the food. Known as nature's scavengers, pigs will eat anything thrown their way, and if that happens to be a pail of slop mixed with manure, they'll go for it.

Notice that I've been charitably referring to these barnyard animals as "pigs." Would pork—the world's most widely eaten meat—be as appetizing if we had to ask the butcher for a slice of swine or several hog chops? I don't think so, even though the National Pork Producers Council drums the saying, "Pork—the other white meat" into our craniums. That takes our minds off the true source of this unclean meat.

I can remember only eating pork one time in my life—some bacon back in high school. My wife, Nicki, feels just as strongly as I do about not eating pork. (You should read what she has to say in *The Great Physician's Rx for Women's Health*, released in 2007.) If you still have trouble with this commandment, try focusing on this one: "Thou shalt not eat anything Jesus cast demons into." I doubt our Lord and Savior would waste thousands of pounds of food.

We feel the same way about shellfish, which is also labeled as "detestable" and "unclean" in Leviticus 11 and Deuteronomy 14. God called hard-shelled crustaceans such as lobsters, crabs, shrimp, and clams unclean because they are bottom feeders that sustain themselves on fish droppings and the dregs of sea life. You've heard the saying that you are what you eat, but when it comes to eating the flesh of shellfish and pigs, you are what *they* ate.

For many of you, the idea of not eating pork, shrimp, and lobster—the Holy Grail of American eating—sounds antisocial, even radical. I remember meeting a young mother, Gidget Stous, who told me that she had an emotional attachment to bacon on her breakfast plate and pork chops with mashed potatoes and gravy for dinner. Her extended family loved barbecue. Yet eating unclean foods fouls the body and introduces toxins into the bloodstream. God declared these meats unclean because He understands the ramifications of eating them, and you should as well.

I strongly urge you and your family to stop eating pork and shellfish. You won't miss them, especially after you replace these unclean meats with delicious grass-fed beef and lamb, as well as wild-caught fish.

Chew on This Advice

I'm starting to sound like my parents every time we eat as a family.

"Joshua, don't forget: chew your food well."

My three-year-old mischievously grins as he shovels another large forkful of Nicki's buffalo meat loaf into his mouth and gulps it down the hatch.

And so the battle goes.

I'm sure my parents got after me to chew my food well before swallowing, but I probably didn't heed their advice any more than Joshua is these days. I'll keep gently reminding my son to chew well, however, because properly masticating food before it's swallowed enhances the digestive process.

Someday, when Joshua's older, I'll explain the biology behind chewing your food well. After you swallow, the food enters your esophagus, the ten-inch-long muscular tube that leads to the stomach. How long the food spends in the esophagus depends on how well it was chewed. Food that has been chewed well makes the journey in just seven seconds. Food that's dry or not properly chewed can take a full minute to make its way through the esophagus, which is not good for the delicate tissues lining this tube between the throat and the stomach. Improperly chewed food that reaches the stomach takes longer to digest, which creates acute, temporary stress on the entire gastrointestinal system.

Chewing foods properly allows enzymes in your children's saliva to turn the food into a near-liquid form before swallowing. The mucous in saliva adheres to food, making it slippery so that the lubricated food can shimmy down the esophagus like a firefighter sliding down a slick pole to answer an emergency call. I recommend that you teach your children to chew each mouthful of food at least twenty to twenty-five times before swallowing.

I know that sounds like a lot of jaw-fatiguing chewing, but just getting them to slow down and not wolf down their food will be a major victory. Although I wasn't much of a chewer as a kid, I've become much better. In fact, if you were to eat with me sometime, you'd be surprised at how long I take to chew my food. I've trained myself to make a conscious effort to chew my food slowly so that plenty of digestive juices are added to the food before it winds through the digestive tract.

Another point: teaching your children to chew slowly and thoroughly will also help them maintain a healthy weight because when they chew their food longer, their brains will receive a signal that they're getting full, so they'll feel satiated earlier.

VI. Thou Shalt Start the Kids' Day with a Healthy Breakfast

One hundred years ago, breakfast for the upper class involved a banquet of steaks, roasts, chops, oysters, and grilled fish accompanied by fried potatoes, scrambled eggs, biscuits, breads, and coffee. The have-nots began the day with a bland fare of porridge, farina, gruel, and other boiled grains.

At the end of the nineteenth century, two brothers, John Harvey Kellogg, M.D., and Will Keith Kellogg, ran the Battle Creek Sanitarium in central Michigan, a prototypical health spa that catered to the wealthy, constipated members of the society pages. Perhaps the uptight rich folks felt bloated from the rich foods and heavy sauces they ate for breakfast.

Dr. John Harvey Kellogg, who ran the sanitarium, was a health nut with a big thing for enemas. He believed a vegetarian diet, coupled with physical exercise and colon cleanses, was the "Road to Wellville," which was the title of a raunchy 1994 Hollywood film about the Battle Creek Sanitarium and Dr. Kellogg.

At any rate, after Dr. Kellogg hooked you up to his enema machine, he flooded your bowel with fifteen gallons of water in a matter of seconds, which got things moving rapidly. Then he directed you to eat half a pint of yogurt. The other half pint was administered you-know-where. The result: a squeaky-clean intestine and all your troubles down the drain.

Will, the younger brother, performed the grunt work at the Battle Creek Sanitarium. He kept the books, bought supplies, answered the mail, and cleaned the bathrooms (which had to be an onerous chore). One day, when Will was making some granola, he left a batch of boiled wheat paste out overnight. The next morning, instead of throwing the dried mixture out, Will ran it through rollers. Out came thin flakes, which Will baked. The Battle Creek clients loved them, and that was the start of the Kellogg cereal company.

The Joke's on Them

Here's a groaner the kids will love:

A man was found dead in his home over the weekend. Detectives called to the scene found the man face down in his bathtub.

The tub had been filled with milk, sugar, and cornflakes. A banana was sticking out of his right ear.

Police suspect a cereal killer . . .

Here's where the story gets interesting: in the early 1900s, the fledgling cereal company was floundering from stiff competition; there were around one hundred cereal companies in Battle Creek alone. Will, looking to sweeten profits, tinkered with the recipe for Corn Flakes by adding cane sugar—normally a forbidden ingredient at the sanitarium. Customers loved the sweetened cereal, sales soared, and the rest is history. Today, breakfast cereal is a mature $9 billion business, and nearly half of the US population eats cold or hot cereal seven days a week. Americans eat 160 bowls per capita each year.

I think you can guess how I feel about commercial breakfast cereal: it's a highly processed, heavily sugared, low-nutrition product that's not part of the recommended foods for *The Great Physician's Rx for Children's Health*. But ol' Will Keith Kellogg must have turned over in his grave when Kellogg's—of all companies—released three new cereals in 2006: Organic Raisin Bran, Organic Rice Krispies, and Organic Mini-Wheats. The boxes are stamped with "USDA Organic," meaning at least 95 percent of the ingredients are organic. These back-to-basics cereals contain no trans fats, no artificial flavors, no artificial sweeteners, no artificial colors, but they are sweetened with evaporated cane juice, so parents beware. While these Kellogg's organic cereals aren't perfect, at least they're a start in the right direction and one more sign that Corporate America is getting it.

I think the best breakfasts, though, aren't built around cold cereal but rather foods like organic eggs, yogurt and fresh fruit, hot oatmeal, or a delicious smoothie. (You can find more than 250 delicious and healthy recipes for breakfast, lunch, and dinner at www.BiblicalHealthInstitute.com.)

Taking the extra time to serve your children a nutritious breakfast will give them a head start in the classroom. Children who eat a healthy breakfast do better in elementary school: they have more alert memories, pay closer attention to the teacher, and visually perceive things better, according to a study published in *Physiology & Behavior*.[32] Eating breakfast speeds up your child's metabolism like cordwood that stokes a fire. He or she will have more energy to burn.

If your children insist on eating their favorite cold cereal, have them mix it with yogurt instead of milk. For hot oatmeal, replace the milk with a pat of butter.

VII. Thou Shalt Pack Healthy School Lunches

Celebrity chef Jamie Oliver of the Discovery Channel cajoled and shamed the British authorities into banning junk food from London school cafeterias and allowing him to come up with economical, healthy lunches that kids would actually eat.

As they say in England, Oliver's twist really started a row.

Out was miserable grub like gristly hamburgers and "chips," or what we call french fries, as well as "Turkey Twizzlers"—miniscule bits of processed meats dusted with bread crumbs and fried in lard. In was healthy fare, like grilled

Starting the Morning Off Right

Can you name the best-selling breakfast cereal in America?

O, let me give you a hint. (That's the hint.)

You're right—*O* as in Cheerios! This toasted oatmeal cereal from General Mills has captured 11 percent of the breakfast cereal market, according to A.C. Nielsen—nearly *three* times that of the next best-selling cereal in America: Kellogg's Frosted Flakes.

That's grrrrreat!

Well, maybe not that great. Popular cereals like Lucky Charms, Cap'n Crunch, and Honey Bunches of Oats aren't the healthiest breakfast fare because they are made from highly processed grains, are high in carbohydrates and added sugar, and may contain preservatives. Sometimes I wonder if kids would be better off nutritionally eating the cardboard box than what's inside.

Okay, so that's an exaggeration, but there's some good news to report: amid much fanfare, General Mills replaced the processed grains with whole grains in their lineup of breakfast cereals. Whole grains are much better for you because they contain fiber and more essential vitamins and minerals. Every nutritionist prefers whole grains over refined grains, which are stripped of their vitamin, mineral, and fiber content during the refining process. These missing nutrients explain why breakfast cereal manufacturers feel compelled to "fortify" their products with vitamins and minerals.

Yet after General Mills introduced whole grains into their cereals, the behemoth company revealed that twenty-eight of the company's fifty-two cereals contained the same level of fiber as before.[33] A total of twenty-two cereals had only one gram of fiber, and five didn't have any fiber at all: Boo Berry, Frosted Chex, Honey Nut Chex, Franken Berry, and Shrek.

I don't think you should have to play a guessing game on whether you're eating a healthy cereal. Although as a general rule I don't eat or recommend dry cereals, my personal favorite is Ezekiel 4:9 cereal, which contains organic sprouted, 100 percent whole wheat; malted barley; organic sprouted barley; organic sprouted millet; organic sprouted lentils; organic sprouted soybeans; organic sprouted spelt; filtered water; and sea salt. Ezekiel 4:9 cereal has a whopping six grams of dietary fiber per serving, which is 24 percent of the daily value for a 2,000 calorie diet.

Now, if the makers of Ezekiel 4:9 cereal can get a tiger or a cap'n behind their cereal . . .

salmon, balsamic beef, fresh mashed potatoes, and fruit salad. Elementary, my dear Watson, except that a vocal minority called the healthy foods "rubbish" and sneaked off during the lunch recess to buy gnarly items like a chip butty, a french-fries-and-butter sandwich doused in vinegar.

The school lunch situation is hardly better on this side of the pond where each day, 50 percent of US school kids eat a cafeteria-provided lunch, which typically consists of two hot dogs in soft, white-bread buns, a half dozen tater tots, a couple of twigs of broccoli and high-fat dip, and homogenized milk or a sugared "fruit drink."[34] This typical lunch meal sounds downright healthy, however, when compared to what a Boston-area grammar school cafeteria offers: "Fluffernutter" sandwiches, a peanut-butter sandwich with an extra layer of Marshmallow Fluff, a locally made, sugary spread.[35]

Like Jamie Oliver, I've been working with several schools outside of Florida to ditch the junk food and actually serve something nutritious. The kids have responded well, and we'll see how this experiment plays out in the future. As for your situation, until school districts overhaul cafeteria menus, I would strongly urge you to make sack lunches for the kids by using organic whole-grain and sprouted breads, peanut or almond butter, whole-grain crackers, fruit, and whatever other healthy foods your children enjoy. You might also want to remind your kids that it might not be a good idea to trade for junk food, like someone I know did twenty years ago.

Pack nutritious snacks, too, because campus vending machines dispense Pepsi, Doritos, Skittles, and caffeinated soft drinks like Mountain Dew, Surge, Josta, and Jolt, which deliver a caffeine punch of 92 milligrams per twenty-ounce drink—the equivalent of a five-ounce cup of brewed coffee. Caffeine causes nervousness, irritability, restlessness, and fidgetiness, which means that teachers must contend with caffeine-hopping kids in their classrooms.

Kids have easy access to these junk foods because hundreds of school districts have made exclusive marketing deals with Pepsi or Coke in the last decade for the exclusive right to sell its sugar-sweetened products in the cafeteria and in vending machines strategically placed around campus (see sidebar on the next page). In exchange, school districts receive up-front fees as well as a commission on sales that can be used to purchase sports equipment or sponsor field trips. I view this as selling out our kids' long-term health for short-term gain.

Fortunately, the pendulum is starting to swing the other way as school administrators do the math: soda pop plus vending machines equals childhood obesity. In 2006, the William J. Clinton Foundation brokered a sweeping deal with Coke, Pepsi, Schweppes, and the American Beverage Association to sell only water, fruit juice, and low-fat milk in elementary and middle schools. Although commercial fruit juice and low-fat milk are problematic, at least some of the people in charge are recognizing an insidious problem on our school campuses.

VIII. Thou Shalt Prepare Healthy Meals for Dinner

Did I just hit a raw nerve?

I thought so.

No meal falls more between the cracks than dinner. Fixing supper falls in the middle of the hectic transition between work and home life, when stress levels are high from running the kids to karate and ballet classes, and fatigue is nipping at the heels. Not to mention how your rambunctious children are ravenous as wolves about this time.

Coming Soon to a School Near You?

From a news article that we might see in the not-so-distant future:

(Los Angeles) The Los Angeles Unified School District, the nation's largest, announced today that Pepsi Cola has won the "naming rights" to its newest charter school that will open next fall in Pomona.

The move came as no surprise to parent-teacher groups and traditionalists who have been fighting the growing trend to name high schools after corporations in recent years.

"With the opening of Pizza Hut High in Pasadena, Chipotle Middle School in Calabassas, and Taco Bell Elementary in Tustin in the last few years, the handwriting was on the wall," said Heather Keener, president of Save Our Schools from Tyrannical Corporations.

LA Unified School District president Reginald Jackson said he understood the parental concerns, but nonetheless, he believed the board's decision was made with the children's best interests in mind.

"In an era when state and federal governments have turned their backs on local education, it was incumbent on us to provide our children with the quality education they need and deserve in the twenty-first century," said Jackson. "Our association with Pepsi is about opportunity, about doing what's right, about benefiting our greatest national treasure—our children."

In exchange for exclusive naming rights to LA Unified School District's newest charter school, district coffers will receive $1 million a year for twenty-five years. "We're not talking vending-machine change," said Jackson. "This is a significant investment from Pepsi on behalf of our children. With this financial shot in the arm, we're hoping that Pepsi High will become a powerhouse school."

Nicki grew up in a home where her mother of three worked full time, and her mantra at dinnertime was: *It has to be quick and easy.* Perhaps that's the way you operate as well. As I mentioned earlier in this chapter, though, relying on chicken nuggets, Tuna Helper, Domino's Pizza, or ready-to-heat meals is not a good way to serve your children foods that God created in a form that's healthy for their bodies.

Preparing dinner from fresh, healthful, organic foods takes planning and effort, but I can't think of a more rewarding chore in terms of your children's physical *and* mental health (see sidebar on page 51). If you're in a time crunch, I suggest that you try a concept called "thrice-a-week" cooking, which means that every time you prepare a hot meal, you make enough of the main dish and the starch to get another dinner out of it. Having extra servings of Nicki's Meatloaf and Mashed Potatoes (just two of the more than 250 delicious and healthy recipes that you'll find at www.BiblicalHealthInstitute.com) can get you out of a jam faster than you can heat these leftovers up in a saucepan lined with extra virgin coconut oil. You can also prepare fresh salads ahead of time by storing washed and torn lettuce in airtight containers or buying prewashed salad mixes.

One Saturday morning, you could brown ten to fifteen pounds of grass-fed hamburger meat and package the cooked meat in one-pound freezer bags. Take a bag or two out in the morning, and when you come back home in the late afternoon, you have the mixings to make tacos, chili, or spaghetti sauce in a matter of minutes. The same advice works for chicken breasts, which can be diced, cooked and browned, and refrigerated for later use as an entrée or in a dinner salad.

It's preferable, however, to cook foods as fresh as possible, and there are plenty of recipes at www.BiblicalHealthInstitute.com to make dinner an anticipated event in your home.

IX. Thou Shalt Drink Water

One of the great convenience food inventions is boxed juice, like Juicy Juice or pouches of Capri Sun Sport. They are viewed by millions of parents as "healthy" alternatives to soft drinks, so into lunch boxes they go.

The Family That Eats Together . . .

. . . . stays healthy together. Columbia University researchers found that the more often a family eats together, the more healthful the foods they eat and the deeper their discussions.[36]

In ways we don't always understand, a shared meal at dinnertime anchors the family and allows the children a forum to express their dreams, their fears, and even their crazy ideas. They pick up new vocabulary and a sense of how conversation should flow.

Children who enjoy regular dinners with their parents have higher academic scores, higher IQs, better vocabularies, nicer manners, greater self-esteem, and fewer problems with smoking, alcohol and drug use, promiscuity, and fighting.[37] Whenever possible, sit down and break bread together.

Kids aren't developing a taste for water if they're sipping straws filled with these sweet "fruit drinks," many of which are flavored with high fructose corn syrup. Most of these beverages contain 10 percent or less of pure fruit juice; the remaining 90 percent is water, sugar, high fructose corn syrup, and additives. If you see words like "drink," "punch," "cocktail," or "beverage" on the product, they're junk.

"Fitness water" like Propel and sports drinks like Gatorade don't meet the Great Physician's standard, either. Propel and other flavored waters are marketed as having fewer calories, less sugar content, and less carbohydrates than Gatorade, but sucrose syrup—a form of sugar—is listed as the second ingredient. So why is sugar being used in a "healthy water"?

As for Gatorade, Powerade, and All Sport, I don't accept their claims that sports drinks rehydrate athletes better than water, an odorless and colorless liquid created by God to regulate body temperature, carry nutrients to the cells, cushion joints, and help young bodies grow. Sports drinks, on the other hand, are man-made combinations of unpurified water, sucrose (table sugar), glucose and fructose syrups, citrus acid, and some potassium and sodium chloride (table salt). Gatorade's salty aftertaste doesn't quench thirst nearly as well as cool spring water, and flavoring and coloring agents are why Gatorade can offer more than two dozen flavors, including Berry Rain, Fierce Wild Berry, and Fruit Punch.

I know kids think it's cooler to drink Lime Rain Gatorade, like their sports heroes, but water is so much better for them that there's no comparison. F. Batmanghelidj, M.D. and author of *You're Not Sick, You're Thirsty!*, says that because children grow like weeds, they are constantly and naturally dehydrated. "The process of cell expansion and division uses up a great deal of water," Dr. Batmanghelidj explains. "Seventy-five percent of each cell is water. The body for a growing child constantly needs and calls for water; otherwise, growth would not be possible. If the natural calls of the body for water are satisfied by manu-factured chemical-containing fluids and sugar-containing drinks, healthy growth and development—events that water itself initiates—may not take place efficiently, and crisis events such as asthma and allergies may occur. Children should learn to drink water by itself and not substitute other beverages."[38]

Water happens to be the perfect fluid replacement; only God could come up with a calorie-free and sugar-free substance that makes up 92 percent of blood plasma and 50 percent of everything else in the body. Water performs many vital tasks for children's growing bodies: regulating body temperature, carrying nutrients and oxygen to the cells, cushioning joints, protecting organs and tissues, and removing toxins.

Children should be drinking a minimum of four to six glasses of water a day; at least double that if they're participating in after-school sports teams and working up a heavy thirst. Again, if your children see *you* sipping on a water bottle throughout the day, they'll be more likely to follow your lead.

One summertime juice I do like is homemade lemonade. I like to mix spring water with fresh lemon juice and honey, which makes for a delicious, hydrating beverage. And in the hot summers, I like to make lemonade slushies by blending ice into the mixture.

A Doctor's Rx: Drink Water!
by Dr. Fiona Blair

When it comes to keeping your children well hydrated, I have the same challenges with my children—it's difficult to get them to drink enough water! What I do at home is make sure my four children each have their own water glass, labeled with his or her name. The goal, I remind them, is to drink half their weight in ounces. For example, my eleven-year-old son, Justin, weighs eighty pounds, so he has to drink forty ounces of water, or five cups, each day.

That's the goal, anyway, and during the sizzling summers in "Hotlanta," they have no problem guzzling tons of water. It's the school months that are more difficult since the strong thirst is not there. But I keep plugging away and set a good example by drinking eight to twelve cups of water a day myself.

Some of the mothers who see me at my office say no matter how hard they try, they can't get their children to drink the water their young bodies need. In those cases, I recommend that parents take a small glass of fruit juice—the good stuff, not something full of sugar—and dilute it with water. With each successive glass, I recommend diluting the fruit juice even more until the child is drinking basically water with a hint of fruit juice.

X. Thou Shalt Not Worry about the Price of Eating Organically

If you live near a Whole Foods store, you may have heard it called "Whole Paycheck" because that's how expensive it is to shop there.

I will concede that organic products cost anywhere from 10 percent to 200 percent more than conventionally produced foods. But as I'm fond of saying on my television show, "You can pay the farmer more now, or you can pay the doctor more later."

But aren't those flaxseed crackers you feed Joshua way more expensive than Cheerios and Goldfish?

Yes, a four-ounce package of flaxseed crackers costs around five bucks, the same amount it costs to purchase a fifteen-ounce box of Cheerios. But what price tag can you put on your child's health? Besides, you can find cheaper organic crackers or snacks if you put your mind to it. As for your weekly food shopping, my best argument is that you can feed your family two or three dinners with organic meats, vegetables, and salad for what it would cost to feed a family of four for one evening at Papa John's Pizza.

While organic foods are more expensive, they're getting cheaper all the time as the volume of shoppers for organic foods grows. Remember, the organic food market has been increasing at an eye-popping 20 percent annual clip in recent years, which means places like Whole Foods and Wild Oats may have to come up with a slogan similar to Wal-Mart's "Watch for Falling Prices."

All-Star Foods

We've discussed many healthy foods in this chapter so far, but now I'd like to share some specific all-stars that you should feeding your children on a regular basis:

1. **Chicken soup.** Joshua didn't wait until four years of age to eat his first piece of meat, like I did. I think we spoon-fed chicken soup to him when he was eight months old. It is one of the best ways to introduce your child to meat. Homemade chicken soup presents your children with soft, well-cooked meat, vegetables, and easily absorbed minerals and gelatin.

Chicken soup, when made by your loving hands, makes for a nutritious meal and a great anti-cold resource when the kids start sniffling. Stephen Rennard, M.D., chief of pulmonary medicine at the University of Nebraska Medical Center in Omaha, says that chicken soup acts as an anti-inflammatory because it apparently reduces the inflammation that occurs whenever coughs and congestion strike respiratory tracts. In addition, chicken soup keeps a check on inflammatory white blood cells, also known as *neutrophils*, which are produced by the onset of cold symptoms.

Dr. Rennard conducted a full-blown study on the medicinal qualities of chicken soup. He had his wife prepared a batch using a recipe from her Lithuanian grandmother. Then he carted the homemade chicken soup to his laboratory, where he combined some of the soup with neutrophils to see what would happen. As Dr. Rennard suspected, his wife's homemade chicken soup demonstrated that neutrophils showed less of a tendency to congregate, but at the same time, these neutrophils did not lose any of their ability to fight off germs, which is a boost for the immune system.[39]

Nicki cooks the best chicken soup ever, based on a recipe inspired by my Grandmother Rose and Sally Fallon, author of *Nourishing Traditions*.

Chicken Soup
Ingredients:

1 whole chicken (free range, pastured, or organic chicken)

2–4 chicken feet (optional)

3–4 quarts cold filtered water

1 tablespoon raw apple cider vinegar

4 medium onions, coarsely chopped

8 carrots, peeled and coarsely chopped

6 celery stalks, coarsely chopped

2–4 zucchinis chopped

4–6 tablespoons extra-virgin coconut oil

1 bunch parsley

5 garlic cloves

1 4-inch piece ginger, grated

2–4 tablespoons Celtic Sea Salt

1/4–1/2 teaspoon cayenne pepper

Directions: If you are using a whole chicken, remove fat glands and the gizzards from the cavity. By all means, use chicken feet if you can find them. Place chicken or chicken pieces in a large stainless steel pot with the water, vinegar, and all vegetables and spices except parsley. Let stand for ten minutes before heating. Bring to a boil and remove scum that rises to the top. Cover and cook for twelve to twenty-four hours. The longer you cook the stock, the more healing it will be. About fifteen minutes before finishing the stock, add parsley. This will impart additional mineral ions to the broth.

Remove from heat and take out the chicken and the chicken feet. Let it cool and remove chicken meat from the carcass, discarding the bones and the feet. Drop the meat back into the soup.

You can make Chicken Soup in a Crock-Pot and let it simmer all day. Leftovers can be used for another meal or weekend lunch.

2. Lamb. Grass-fed lamb, the meat of young sheep less than a year old, is a biblical meat extraordinaire (see Exodus 29). In addition, lamb is an excellent source of protein, zinc, and vitamin B_{12}, and has three times more heart-healthy omega-3 fatty acids, the so-called "good fats," than other meats, and contains conjugated linoleic acid (CLA) and carnitine. Sometimes I wish we lived in New Zealand, where fifty-six million sheep outnumber the human population by a ratio of 16 to 1![40]

I've already extolled the virtues of eating grass-fed lamb earlier in this chapter, but I urge you to look for more ways to get this sweet, tender, and complexly flavored meat on your dining room table.

3. Sheep's milk yogurt. It may sound like we're staying in the same *Jeopardy* category here, but the thick, silky texture and mellow, creamy taste of sheep's milk yogurt is a healthy and delicious alternative to commercial yogurt from factory farms. Sheep's milk yogurt has up to twice the calcium as cow's or goat's milk yogurt, more than triple the vitamin D, and up to four times the amount of medium-chain triglycerides and muscle-building whey protein. My favorite brand of sheep's milk yogurt is Old Chatham, which is available at local health food stores.

4. High omega-3 eggs. Up to this point, I haven't mentioned eggs, which have gotten a bad rap in recent years for being a high-fat, high-cholesterol food. Yet high omega-3 eggs, when consumed from free-range and organic sources, contain fats that young bodies need to grow up big and strong.

The humble egg is a wonderful food deserving Hall of Fame status. This nutrient-dense food packs six grams of protein, a bit of vitamin B_{12}, vitamin E, lutein, riboflavin, folic acid, calcium, zinc, iron, and essential fatty acids into a mere seventy-five calories. I strongly urge you to scramble, poach, hard-boil, or cook with high omega-3 eggs, which have become much more available in response to rising consumer demand. Natural food markets stock them, of course, but you'll also find high omega-3 eggs at major supermarket chains as well as warehouse clubs like Costco. Omega-3 egg yolk was Joshua's first solid food at six months of age.

5. Porridge. When I was eight years old, the Village Players theater group in Palm Beach announced an open casting call for their theatrical production of *Oliver!* I won the role of Oliver, the orphan boy who runs away from a London orphanage and falls in with a gang of boy thieves run by the wizard of pickpocketry, Fagin.

I remember pretending to eat a lot of porridge during the play's eight-performance run. I understand that porridge is an antiquated word redolent of Dickens and Victorian England, but porridge can be made from just about any grain that has been hulled and mechanically broken in some manner. These grains are cooked in water until soft. In America, we generally call this oatmeal, which is available in rolled, steel-cut, and stone-ground versions. Oatmeal is enjoying a revival these days.

Oats are a concentrated source of fiber and nutrients that contain healthy compounds called *beta glucans*, which enhance the immune system and promote healthy blood sugar levels. Beta glucans encourage the growth of good bacteria in the digestive system and substantially lower the risk of type 2 diabetes, which is becoming more and more common among overweight children. Serve porridge—or organic oatmeal—with a pat of butter instead of milk, and go ahead and add a spoonful of organic maple syrup to sweeten it. Keep in mind that the best oatmeal often needs thirty minutes to cook and soften.

I make a seven-to-nine grain porridge from grains that I grind myself. I then soak everything overnight in water to enhance digestion. Upon rising, I add more water and cook the mixture on the stove. Once my oatmeal is ready, I add butter, cinnamon, raisins, and honey. This makes for an awesome breakfast, especially in wintertime.

6. Sprouted or yeast-free bread. Listen, I love bread. Nicki and I have been fortunate to travel to Europe a couple of times, and one of the taste treats of the Old Country has been chewing on a crunchy piece of Parisian sourdough or a whole grain Italian flat bread called *ciabatta.*

When we're back Stateside, though, standard-issue white bread doesn't quite cut it for us. Commercial bread is a highly processed commodity that packs the same nutrition power as sawdust, which pretty much sums up the lousy taste of white and so-called "wheat" bread. One of the dirty little secrets of today's commercial wheat bread is that it only looks brown because it's colored with caramel. The main ingredient of white *and* wheat bread is white enriched flour, which is a highly allergenic, difficult-to-digest substance that's been stripped of all the "good stuff"—vitamins and minerals—and mixed with emulsifiers, artificial chemicals, and hydrogenated oils containing trans fats. *Blelch!*

Breads made from sprouted or yeast-free wheat are a nutritional night-and-day difference. Most major supermarkets carry sprouted and yeast-free whole grain breads in their frozen section. As you would expect, you can also find these healthy breads at a natural foods store, or you can make your own with a bread machine.

7. Avocados. One of the great things about living in Florida is our access to inexpensive avocados. We find ourselves adding creamy, rich slices of avocado to our salads, eggs, and salsa and just about any other food that we can make an excuse for. Avocados have gotten a bad rap for being high in fat—"butter pears," they're called—but they contain "good" monounsaturated fats that lower cholesterol levels. Researchers have discovered that avocados are rich in beta-sitosterol, a natural substance shown to significantly lower blood cholesterol numbers.

8. Berries. I love any fruit that ends with the suffix *berries:* blueberries, raspberries, blackberries, huckleberries, cranberries, and strawberries. Brimming with cell-protecting antioxidants, berries make great snacks because of their sweet but tart flavors. Your favorite berries are the key ingredients for smoothies that can make a meal or a dessert. Warehouse clubs like Costco sell big bags of frozen organic berries at reasonable prices, although you can never beat a flat of fresh berries in season.

Berries are great in smoothies, muffins, salads, and as a dessert topped with organic whipped cream. Joshua, when he was two, would often eat two cups of blueberries, strawberries, and raspberries at one sitting.

9. Bananas. *Kids go bananas over bananas.* Seems like there's a song there, but kids love bananas because they contain natural sugars as well as fiber and potassium. Bananas also contain *tryptophan*, a type of protein that the body converts into serotonin, which improves moods. Here's a delicious, elliptically shaped, yellow fruit that's readily available anytime as a "fast food."

10. Coconut pudding. I'm not talking about making coconut pudding from store-bought mixes, but organic coconut pudding made with the meat of young coconuts and mixed in a high-speed blender with honey, vanilla, and even organic cocoa powder. Now, there's a great-tasting dessert. Coconuts, which contain significant amounts of health-promoting medium-chain fatty acids, increase levels of beneficial HDL or "good" cholesterol.

I'm not boasting when I say my coconut chocolate mousse pudding is to die for or, better yet, live for. (You can find the recipe at www.BiblicalHealth Institute.com.)

11. Organic whole food nutrition bars. Energy bars are marketed as a nutritious, candy-bar-sized alternative to Snickers. In many ways, energy bars are the perfect snacks to hold kids over when you're doing errands in the minivan.

No longer a niche product for endurance athletes, energy bars have gone mainstream. Sales have doubled in the last couple of years, a palpable demonstration that energy bars have gotten better tasting in recent years. "Convenience bars" no longer taste like the morning newspaper; today, you can choose from flavors that appeal to the sweet tooth: Fudge Graham, Chocolate Peanut Butter, and Devil's Food Cake, to name a few. They really do taste like a Snickers, except for a certain aftertaste. So are they healthy?

I think you already know my answer: most energy bars are not the nutritional powerhouses they are purported to be. At the end of the day, many energy bars are nothing more than glorified candy bars: a highly processed mix of protein powders (soy or milk), sugars and/or artificial sweeteners, chemicals, preservatives, and synthetic ingredients. If it looks like a candy bar, tastes like a candy bar, and has many of the same ingredients as a candy bar . . . then it's a candy bar.

All is not lost, however. Some excellent organic nutrition bars have hit the market recently, including food bars that I personally formulated after three years of development. Garden of Life Living Food bars are certified organic, high in fiber and antioxidants, and contain gut-friendly probiotics. Garden of Life Living Food Bars are made from whole foods, including raw honey, almond butter, organic fruits, sprouted whole grains, and beta glucans from soluble oat fiber. They come in four delicious flavors: Perfect Food Raspberry Green, Chocolate Coated Perfect Food, Summer Berry Antioxidant, and Apple Cinnamon SuperSeed. These wonderful whole food nutrition bars are perfect for school lunches or afternoon snacks, and the adults I know love them too. You can learn more by visiting www.GardenofLife.com.

EAT: WHAT FOODS ARE EXTRAORDINARY, AVERAGE, OR TROUBLE?

I've prepared a comprehensive list of foods that are ranked in descending order based on their health-giving qualities. Foods at the top of the list are healthier than those at the bottom. The best foods to serve your children are what I call "Extraordinary," which God created for us to eat and will give you and your children the best chance to live long and happy lives. It would be best to serve these foods from the extraordinary category more than 50 to 75 percent of the time.

Foods in the Average category should make up less than 50 percent of your daily diets. Foods in the Trouble category should be served with extreme caution to your children. Better yet, don't buy these foods at all.

For a complete listing of Extraordinary, Average, and Trouble Foods, visit www.BiblicalHealthInstitute.com.

In addition, you can go online at www.foodnews.org and download the Environmental Working Group's wallet-sized Shopper's Guide, which lists the "Dirty Dozen" (the twelve fruits and veggies that are the most contaminated with pesticides) and the "Cleanest 12" (those that generally have the lowest amounts of pesticides).

If you're curious about the ratings, here they are:

The Dirty Dozen
- peaches
- apples
- sweet bell peppers
- celery
- nectarines
- strawberries
- cherries
- pears
- grapes (imported)
- spinach
- lettuce
- potatoes

The Cleanest 12
- onions
- avocados
- sweet corn (frozen)
- pineapples
- mangoes
- asparagus
- sweet peas (frozen)
- kiwifruit
- bananas
- cabbage
- broccoli
- papaya

℞ THE GREAT PHYSICIAN'S Rx FOR CHILDREN'S HEALTH: TEACH THEM TO EAT TO LIVE

- *Serve only foods God created.*

- *Serve only foods in a form healthy for the body.*

- *Shop in natural food stores or the natural and organic section of your grocery store for organic meats, produce, and dairy products.*

- *Eat more grass-fed lamb and sheep's milk yogurt.*

- *Introduce your children to goat's milk cheese and sheep's milk cheese in salads.*

- *Stop preparing yucky meats like pork, shrimp, crab, and lobster.*

- *Read food labels in a search for processed ingredients, artificial flavors, and preservatives.*

- *Wean the kids off fast food.*

- *Make the effort to cook a fresh, hot meal for dinner.*

- *Ban soft drinks and serve water (preferably not from the tap) or 100 percent fruit drinks.*

- *Remind your children to chew their food well—and slow down yourself, too.*

- *Place limits on television, and stick to them, especially on Saturday mornings.*

- *Look at eating organically as a worthy investment in your children's future.*

Take Action

To learn how to incorporate the principles
of nutritious eating into your family, please turn
to page 176 for the Great Physician's Rx for
Children's Health Seven-Day Plan.

KEY #2

Supplement Their Diets
with Whole Food Nutritional Supplements

I t's amazing how advertising jingles stay with you for a long, long time.

I grew up watching my share of Saturday morning cartoons, and as I thought of a way to get into this chapter on nutritional supplements, my mind instantly recalled a tune that I hadn't hummed in years:

We are the Flintstone kids,
Ten million strong . . . and growing!

The jingle that leaped into my brain emanated from a string of Flintstone vitamin commercials that ran in the '80s and are still in rotation today. If your kids park themselves in front of Nickelodeon some morning, sooner or later they'll view one of these catchy, colorful Flintstone ads, which often present the following storyboard:

- Opening scene: young, cherubic voices singing, "*We are the Flintstone kids . . .*" as a pair of cuter-than-custard preschoolers tromps through a sunshiny backyard garden.
- While the kids cavort among cornstalks and tomato plants, a smooth announcer's voice intones, "To help kids get the important vitamins they need, pediatricians know that good nutrition is key. Flintstones Complete Multivitamins in chewable tablets, the pediatrician's number-one choice for healthy, growing kids."
- Closing jingle: *Ten million strong . . . and growing!*

Flintstone Complete vitamins come in fire-engine red boxes with child-proof plastic bottles. Each bottle contains brightly colored, cartoon character–shaped tablets featuring two lovable animated Stone Age families—Fred, Wilma, and Pebbles Flintstone, and their pet dinosaur, Dino; and Barney, Betty, and Bamm-Bamm Rubble—in various fruit flavors. The subliminal message to parents: just hand your little Bamm-Bamm a sweet-tasting Flintstones multivitamin, complete with twelve vitamins and seven minerals, and your prized child will receive the essential nutrients he or she needs to grow up big and strong.

These beguiling ads have sucked in many a parent, including Melissa, a mom writing on Epinions.com:

> Ever since my oldest children were preschoolers, I've been purchasing these Flintstone's Complete Multivitamin, Chewable Tablets as an extra "insurance policy"... since, like most American kids, they don't always eat the right foods all the time. My oldest son... is a very picky eater and would live off pizza and bread if I'd let him, so it makes me feel better knowing that he's getting at least some of the important vitamins and minerals for proper growth and development... He refuses to consume milk and many other calcium rich foods, so even the 10 percent RDA he gets with these is better than nothing. While I know it's best for children to get most of their nutrients from their diet, I realistically know this isn't always happening, so for my own peace of mind... these vitamin and mineral supplements in three flavors with all the classic *Flintstone* characters are the best choice for my family.[1]

I hate to rain on Melissa's parade, but Flintstone chewables don't have me yelling "Yabba-dabba-do" for several reasons, beginning with how they're marketed as vitamin-enriched candy. The Flintstone characters get their sweet flavor from aspartame, a chemical additive and artificial sweetener that you shouldn't give to your child because of the potential long-term health implications.

Furthermore, nutritional supplements shouldn't be viewed as a sweet-tasting "insurance policy" that Mom hands out like a postmeal treat. I've heard reports of preschoolers gobbling up the entire Flintstone family when Mom wasn't looking, which isn't a good idea since the recommended dose is one tablet a day. My biggest concern, however, is that Flintstone vitamins—as well as nearly all the "one-a-day" and commercial supplements sold in supermarkets and vitamin shops today—are produced from isolated or synthetically made nutrients.

For example, the vitamins C and E in nearly all supplements are synthetic forms of the "real" vitamins C and E and don't come from natural sources. What's happened is that biochemists in white lab coats have, over the last few decades, discovered ways to efficiently and inexpensively manufacture these vitamins synthetically by isolating nutrients that sport the same chemical signatures as various vitamins but skip the entire process of nature.

I'll have more to say about this trend shortly, but that doesn't diminish the importance—or my passion—regarding supplementing your children's diets with whole food nutritional supplements, the second key to unlocking your children's health potential.

Chewing on Chewable Vitamins

Kid-friendly chewable vitamins are only as good as what makes them taste good. Many of the popular vitamins for kids, like L'il Critters Gummy Vites and Animal Parade, contain high fructose corn syrup, sucrose, and fructose, which is basically sugar. Don't get me started on vitamins containing artificial flavors or artificial sweeteners like aspartame.

One of the sweeteners I can live with is xylitol, a sugar alcohol that is a white crystalline substance that looks and tastes like sugar. Xylitol can actually be good for teeth and gums and has been shown to reduce tooth decay, so supplements with xylitol would be good to look at.

Not a Replacement

I don't think Flintstone vitamins—or any other form of nutritional supplementation—allow Mom or Dad a free pass for not serving foods created by

God and as close to the natural source as possible. You must still cook and prepare a wide variety of organic foods to meet your kids' nutritional needs and give their growing bodies the key nutrients they need to build strong bones and muscles. You can't let them eat nothing but pizza and bread and expect a bottle of pills to save the day.

At the same time, though, Melissa has a point: kids aren't receiving the important vitamins and minerals they need from the foods they eat, and that's true even for youngsters who enjoy the benefits of an all-organic, all-natural diet. In this day and age, our fruits, grains, and vegetables are harvested from nutrient-deficient soils lacking many of the enzymes, minerals, and micro-organisms found in the soil fifty or one hundred years ago. This systematic hijacking of soil-depleted farmlands is reflected in our supermarkets' produce sections: green tomatoes, tasteless grapes, rock-hard peaches, and limp lettuce. Our grains, no matter how "whole" they're purported to be, are nutritional weaklings when compared to the robust crops of yesteryear.

In addition to the lackluster nutrients found in our food supply, there's another aspect worth noting, and it's that our modern-day diets are seriously low in omega-3 fatty acids and seriously high in omega-6 fatty acids. You may be scratching your head and wondering, *What are omega-3 or omega-6 fatty acids, Jordan?* Answer: they are a group of polyunsaturated fats—also known as essential fatty acids (EFAs)—crucial for a child's normal growth and development as well as brain function. These "good fats" cannot be manufactured naturally in their bodies but must be obtained from the foods they eat. A mother's breast milk contains these fatty acids, but the amount depends on Mom's eating habits.

Omega-3 fatty acids come in three types: alpha linolenic acid (ALA), which is found in flaxseed, walnuts, pumpkin seeds, and hemp seeds; and eicosapen-taenoic acid (EPA) and docosahexaenoic acid (DHA), which are long-chain fatty acids found in cold-water fish and eggs from chickens that run around pecking at worms. Omega-6 fatty acids are found in common vegetables oils: corn oil, safflower oil, sunflower oil, and soybean oil, which are base ingredients in margarine, breads, pastas, baked goods, salad dressings, and a zillion other pack-aged foods.

Omega-3 and omega-6 fatty acids can be called "good fats" as long as they are consumed in the right balance, but there's broad medical agreement that our culture's reliance on processed foods tilts the ratio toward an unhealthy ratio between omega-6s and omega-3s. The proper ratio should be four units of omega-6 fatty acids for every unit of omega-3 (for a ratio of 4 to 1), but researchers say our heavy consumption of processed grains and commercial foods manufactured from vegetable oils means that most of us eat an unhealthy 20-to-1 ratio of omega-6 fatty acids to omega-3 fatty acids.

Such an imbalance triggers all sorts of diseases and unhealthy conditions. For example, excess omega-6 is stored in the body as fat, which is a major reason why we are dealing with childhood obesity today. Over the long term, too much omega-6 raises blood pressure, which leads to blood clots that can instigate heart attacks and strokes.

The best way to improve the omega-6 to omega-3 ratio is to raise the consumption of omega-3 fatty acids, which always come from foods that God created. This is problematic, however, since most children don't eat eggs laid by healthy chickens, don't have a taste for oily fish, and don't snack on flaxseed crackers, all resulting in a significant deficiency in these omega-3 fatty acids. The best solution I've come across is to supplement your children's diets with one of the best sources of essential fatty acids found in nature: cod liver oil. One or two teaspoons a day, depending on their ages and the amount of sunlight they receive, will drastically improve their omega-6 to omega-3 ratios and deliver the essential fatty acids their young bodies need to develop their brains and nervous systems.

Brain Food

Omega-3 fatty acids are essential to brain development because the brain is more than 60 percent structural fat, writes Theresa Gallagher on the Mercola.com Web site.[2] Just as your children's muscles need protein and their bones call for calcium, their developing brains require the essential fats found in omega-3 fatty acids. Approximately 20 percent of the dry weight of the brain and approximately 30 percent of the retina is made from these elements.

Cod liver oil is *the* most important supplement parents can give their progeny. (Fish oil is acceptable, but I prefer cod liver oil.) I've been taking cod liver oil daily for more than a decade and greatly believe in its health-giving properties. Plenty of folks have informed me that cod liver oil has helped them with their failing eyesight, memory problems, and muscle strains. When I formulated Joshua's formula when he was three months old, I knew the *first* nutrient I wanted to include was cod liver oil because of its high concentration of omega-3 fatty acids and vitamins A and D, all nutrients found in a mother's breast milk. Vitamin A is extremely important to the development of the gastrointestinal tract and lungs of children and is three times more prevalent in cod liver oil than beef liver, the next richest source. Vitamin D keeps bones healthy and plays a vital role in immunity and blood cell formation.

Boning Up on Vitamin D

Have you ever thought about how God knew exactly what He was doing when He created our bones? Hard but flexible, lightweight but tough, our bone structure forms a solid but malleable skeleton that gives our bodies definition and strength yet the mobility to move on a dime. The outer layer of our bones is a honeycomb-like material wrapped around hollow pipes that allows for the passage of nutrients and waste. Bone is living tissue that changes constantly, with bits of old bone being removed and replaced by new bone.

Childhood is the most important period of growth for the 206 bones in kids' young bodies. The bones grow the fastest during the first three years of life and because strong bones build strong bodies, pediatricians and nutritionists remind parents to make sure that their children receive enough calcium and vitamin D. The latter nutrient, Vitamin D, aids in the absorption of calcium, which makes it a crucial nutrient for bone health. I'm sure you've seen the compelling "Got Milk?" advertisements on TV and in magazines, featuring celebrities with milk moustaches and a testimonial touting the vitamin D qualities of dairy products.

What doctors and celebrities fail to mention, though, is that vitamin D is only available in relatively small amounts from calcium-rich foods like milk, fish, liver, and egg yolks. Since nearly all children eat these foods in low quantities and don't get much sunshine, especially in northern climates (sunshine is an excellent source of vitamin D, as I'll explain in Key #5), your sons and daughters have a strong chance of being vitamin D deficient.

This is where cod liver oil can come to the rescue. With its chart-topping levels of vitamin D, cod liver oil will help your children grow up with vigorous, healthy bones, which is yet another compelling reason to add this superstar supplement to their diets. Don't confuse cod liver oil with *castor* oil, however, which from early American times to the early twentieth century was often administered to unruly children as a disciplinary measure. Castor oil was the Victorian-era equivalent of Ex-Lax, which leaves me curious why parents would punish their children with a laxative, but I didn't live in those times.

At any rate, more and more research is being done these days on the healthful benefits of cod liver oil, which was popularized 150 years ago in fishing communities dotting the North Atlantic coastlines of Norway, Scotland, and Iceland. During their long, frigid winters, with little fresh food and even less sunlight, pioneering doctors discovered that cod liver oil warded off rickets in malnourished children. Rickets, a childhood disease characterized by defective bone growth, is caused by a lack of vitamin D in the body. Hundreds of years ago, more children suffered from deformed bones than you would think, and unfortunately rickets is enjoying a bit of a resurgence today, as Dr. Blair discusses on the next page.

A Ruckus about Rickets
by Dr. Fiona Blair

You would think that rickets is one of those nineteenth-century diseases that we eradicated a long time ago, but I'm seeing a resurgence of rickets in my practice.

I blame several factors. The first is that children don't drink real milk anymore. Instead of setting whole, raw, or nonhomogenized milk out at the dinner table, mothers ply them with fruit juice, colas, and sports drinks—or the milk they drink is fat-free, which is deficient in vitamin D, a fat-soluble vitamin. Children aren't eating enough fatty fish or egg yolks from free-range chickens either, which are both great sources of essential fatty acids as well as vitamin D.

Another reason I'm seeing more rickets is because ob-gyns and pediatricians have been negligent by not telling mothers to supplement their children's diets or their own diets with vitamin D–rich supplements like cod liver oil. Infants need vitamin D, which they can get from mother's milk as long as the mother gets enough vitamin D. Infants who are bottle-fed can benefit by supplementing with both omega-3 fatty acids as well as vitamin D, which are supplied in abundance in cod liver oil.

Another thing to keep in mind, if you're an African-American, is that your babies are more susceptible to rickets because the melanin in the skin blocks out the sun rays necessary for the body to make its own vitamin D. Finally, babies born in the wintertime, babies born to breast-feeding Muslim mothers (who often cover themselves, thus blocking sun exposure), and breast-feeding mothers who spend a lot of time indoors, are raising children at risk for rickets.

So parents, do three things: give your children omega-3 cod liver oil, feed them fatty fish, and get them out in the sun during the off-peak hours.

These days, though, rickets isn't a major source of worry for parents because there's plenty to eat. Actually, we have a different kind of problem. Because many children eat processed foods for three square meals a day plus sugary snacks, they are beset by too much omega-6 fatty acids circulating in their young, growing bodies. Cod liver oil, with its high levels of omega-3 fatty acids, counteracts that surge, which is why it is one of your biggest weapons against childhood obesity and many other health challenges as your kids grow into adulthood. Furthermore, the omega-3 fatty acid DHA has shown promise for its ability to reduce body fat, according to researchers at the University of Georgia, who believe fatty acids increase the ability of cell membranes to use up blood glucose, meaning there is less left over for the body to turn into excess fat.[3]

Unfortunately for parents, the yellowish oil harvested from the livers of North Atlantic codfish doesn't have Tony the Tiger bellowing "Tastes grrrrrreat!" You may be wondering how you can get your kids—who balk at eating broccoli—to try something as fishy-smelling as cod liver oil.

I understand that some kids will flip their gag switches as soon as you reach for a bottle of cod liver oil from the pantry. But there are ways to make the medicine go down. For infants and toddlers, cod liver oil mixes so well in my infant and toddler formulas (see pages 35–36) that they shouldn't fuss at all. As they grow out of their bottles, you can get creative with a blender by mixing cod liver oil with fruit, kefir, yogurt, or coconut milk.

These days I give Joshua Olde World Icelandic Cod Liver Oil by Garden of Life, which I formulated, the old-fashioned way—right off the spoon. I tell Joshua that taking his cod liver oil will make him big and strong, smart and fast. Judging from his stellar well baby visits to the doctor, preschool report cards, and forty-yard dash time, I think it's working. That spoken from a truly proud papa.

I don't even have to give him a spoonful of sugar to help the cod liver oil go down the hatch. He's fine with the taste because he's probably drunk six thousand bottles of infant and toddler formula with cod liver oil (two and a half years times an average of six bottles of formula per day.) Joshua consumed toddler formula until he was three because I doubted I could ever get this quality of nutrients into his system through diet alone.

Besides, cod liver oil is much more palatable these days, thanks to innovation. You can find Garden of Life's lemon- and mint-flavored cod liver oil in health food stores everywhere. You'll be surprised by the dramatically reduced fishy smell and aftertaste.

A Superstar Supplement
by Dr. Fiona Blair

I like what Jordan has to say about cod liver oil because this nutritional supplement is one of my favorite substances, too. I can usually persuade parents to give it to their children during the winter months to ward off colds and keep the immune system strong, but their enthusiasm seems to wane during the hot summer months here in the South. That's too bad because cod liver oil should be taken year-round since children need an abundant source of omega-3 fats and vitamins A and D every single day of the year, not just during the flu season.

I also recommend cod liver oil to my expectant mothers, as well as those breast-feeding their infants, because of its rich content of high omega-3 fatty acids. Even the makers of commercial formula, such as Similac and Enfamil, have jumped on the omega-3 bandwagon by adding DHA and EPA to their formula lines. These companies refer to the same studies on brain development to state their claims that their formulas can help improve a child's visual acuity and cognitive ability.

Now, if you happen to be pregnant or are nursing a young one, you should be aware that taking cod liver oil can boost their IQs and make them smarter. Seriously.

I know this sounds like something a traveling snake-oil salesman would promise—*Step right up, you ladies with child or nursing a little one. I've got a sure-fire method that will raise their intellectual quotients, and it's right here in this bottle!*

Yet Norwegian researchers conducting a randomized, double-blind trial of

Watch for the Rancid Stuff

Many parents are unaware that cod liver oil—like one of my favorite movie characters, Superman—suffers from a kryptonite-like weakness: rancidity. This nutritional supplement can spoil over time if left exposed to air and heat. Purchase cod liver oil that comes in small bottles of dark glass; then store in a cool, dark place. There's no need to refrigerate cod liver oil if you and your children finish the bottle within a few months.

expectant mothers and those nursing their newborns found that the children whose mothers received cod liver oil scored significantly higher (a little more than four points) on standardized intelligence tests than those whose mothers received corn oil during the same period. The children had their IQs tested when they were four years old, according to *Pediatrics* magazine, which published the study conducted by the Institute for Nutrition Research at the University of Oslo.[4]

Since Nicki faithfully took her cod liver oil during pregnancy and lactation—and I later mixed it into thousands of bottles of formula—I'm expecting Joshua to bring home straight-*A* report cards when he starts school. Nothing less will be acceptable.

I'm kidding, of course, but another point worth noting from this study is that these moms were fed either cod liver oil (which is high in omega-3s) or corn oil (which is high in omega-6s), which further illustrates the importance of the omega-6 to omega-3 ratios that we discussed earlier in this chapter.

Why is cod liver oil so good for cogitation? As it turns out, the DHA in cod liver oil and other fish oils is a "brain food" for developing and growing young minds. According to a study funded by the National Institute of Child Health and Human Development (NICHD), infants who received DHA in supplemental form performed better when it came to skills such as problem solving and memory tests.[5]

Expect to Be Expecting?

Over the years I've been approached by hundreds of women who've asked me what kind of nutritional supplements they should take during their nine-month pregnancy. My recommendation starts with cod liver oil, as you would expect, plus a good whole food multivitamin that's high in folic acid.

If you're having trouble conceiving, my advice would be to cut your consumption of carbohydrates, particularly sugar and starches. In other words, if you have a thing for Starbucks Caramel Macchiatos, like Nicki did, you might want to cut those out. Doing so will help balance your hormonal levels and monthly cycle, giving you the best chance to have normal ovulation.

On the flip side, though, a lack of omega-3 essential fatty acids in their bloodstreams means that kids are more likely to have learning disorders and be hyperactive, according to a Purdue University study.[6] David Horrobin, a medical and biochemical researcher, once said, "If you want to prevent learning disabilities in your children, feed them cod liver oil."[7]

When sober-minded school authorities in Durham, England, noticed that their students had trouble concentrating in the classroom, they started a "programme," as they say in the United Kingdom. Those with learning, behavior, and coordination difficulties were asked to participate in a six-month study: some were given fish oil capsules with DHA and EPA; others in the control group received placebos. Motor skills, reading, spelling, memory, drawing, and handwriting were measured and evaluated.

In typical understated British fashion, the response was "encouraging," said Madeleine Portwood, the senior educational psychologist who ran the trial. Actually, Ms. Portwood should have been ecstatic: in broad terms, the school district saw reading gains of between eighteen months and four years, and

Don't Use a Spoonful of Sugar

Perhaps your children have outgrown bottled formula but are too young to swallow capsules. What are some other ways they can receive their cod liver oil?

As mentioned, smoothies work quite well, but getting out the blender, dicing fruit, and whipping up a thick smoothie can be a time-consuming chore as you're getting them ready for school. Another idea is to mix cod liver oil in their favorite yogurt or kefir. You could try orange juice, but the oily consistency may take some getting used to.

attention gains of as much as 400 percent.[8] The Durham results mirror another omega-3 supplement trial at Cricket Green School in Merton, England, where giving fish oil supplements to schoolchildren resulted in a 5.6 percent reduction in impulsive behavior, a 9.3 percent reduction in inattention, and similar reductions in hyperactivity and social problems.[9]

Cod liver oil is good for your child in ways that we're still discovering. I urge you to introduce this foundational supplement to your children. If you're expecting an addition to the family, then please consume this nutritional supplement while your baby grows and develops in the womb.

Switching Gears

When cardiothoracic surgeon Mehmet Oz, M.D., coauthor of the popular *You: The Owner's Manual,* mentioned probiotics on *Oprah,* the famous daytime television host stopped him and said, "Pro-by-*what?*"

Which only goes to show you that a lot of people haven't heard of probiotics, including the knowledgeable Oprah Winfrey.

Probiotics, by definition, are living microflora that play a critical role in your children's health by supporting normal bowel function and a healthy immune system. Probiotics are "good germs" that the body needs to fend off illness and disease because every gastrointestinal system contains hundreds of different species of various bacteria, otherwise known as *intestinal flora*.

I understand that most parents are more aware of the term *antibiotics* because that's what pediatricians routinely use to treat your children's ear infections or fight off secondary infections caused by their nasty colds and bouts of flu. Antibiotics inhibit the growth of—or destroy—harmful bacteria, but they also nuke good bacteria as well. Antibiotics have been called "wonder drugs" since their discovery in the 1930s because of their ability to cure bacteria-related illnesses such as pneumonia, tuberculosis, and meningitis—deadly diseases that have killed millions of children throughout history. So if *anti*biotics have a well-deserved reputation for saving lives and curing ear infections, does that mean *pro*biotics could open the door to your son or daughter being attacked by a host of childhood illnesses?

Not at all. In fact, your children *need* probiotics because they promote the growth of beneficial microorganisms in their tender tummies. Without these living organisms circulating in their digestive tracts, your children would be susceptible to a wide range of intestinal ailments that could lead to serious digestive-related problems, like Crohn's disease, ulcerative colitis, and gastritis—conditions that often start presenting themselves in the late teen and early adult years. Giving your school-age children probiotics *today* may even save them from the horrible pain of digestive problems *later*.

I'm particularly keen on probiotics because of my own digestive issues that started at age nineteen. I had just finished my freshman year at Florida State University, where I drank from everything that college life had to offer. Besides taking a full load of classes, I participated in several take-life-to-the-max extracurricular activities. I loved singing with a college ministry that reached out to others and performed concerts at churches along the Florida panhandle. I won a spot on the Florida State cheerleading squad shortly after I arrived on campus, so that meant practicing every day after class and leading cheers on football and basketball weekends. I proudly wore my garnet-and-gold FSU sweater and pleated pants while exhorting the student section to fire up the 'Noles. With so much going on, schoolwork became almost an afterthought.

Keeping up with my classes and doing my homework—difficult because I've never been a voracious reader—proved to be a challenge. I blew off steam by playing intramural football during my "free" time.

Then—like a haymaker punch in the stomach—digestive problems hit me full force. As I detail in *The Great Physician's Rx for Health and Wellness*, my digestive troubles landed me in the hospital, and I'll never forget the dark evening when I heard one of my hospital nurses whispering to another that she didn't think I'd survive the night. I rallied, however, but I didn't make a full recovery from my two-year health odyssey until I added various probiotics to my diet, which improved the microbial balance in my gastrointestinal tract.

If you have not been serving your family foods that God created, there's a better-than-even chance that your children—especially if they are nearing adolescence—have an imbalance of microflora in their guts. This condition, known medically as *dysbiosis*, is often caused by the overconsumption of antibiotics, a diet high in processed and refined foods, and a lack of beneficial microorganisms in the diet. Probiotics can swing the pendulum back in the other direction.

You can make sure your children receive their probiotics in one of two ways: food or dietary supplements. Health food stores, as well as more and more supermarkets, stock probiotic-rich yogurt and kefir. The next time you pass the refrigerated dairy case, notice how many of the yogurt and kefir products tout probiotics on their packaging.

While serving your children yogurt and kefir made from organic sources is commendable, there are dietary supplements just for children that will introduce beneficial microorganisms to their digestive tracts, which does several very healthy things: improve bowel and immune system function, increase the absorption of nutrients from the foods they eat, and eliminate toxins from their bodies.

Probiotics available in kid-friendly powder form can be readily mixed in smoothies or added to certain foods. Be sure to look for probiotics formulated to provide the flora found naturally in a child's digestive system, meaning it contains fewer strains of probiotics than those marketed for adults. One of the ingredients to look for is *Saccharomyces boulardii*, a friendly yeast that supports

When's the Best Time?

The best time to give your children nutritional supplements is in the morning or evening. If your children are school age, don't forget that they can't bring any supplements to school. In these "zero-tolerance" days, gulping down pills during recess or lunch—no matter how healthy they are—is a nonstarter.

There is a convenient way to get probiotics into your child's belly during school, however. I recommend packing their lunch boxes with organic yogurt or kefir, if they can put their lunch in a refrigerator when they arrive at school. Since refrigeration isn't usually available, you could also pack Garden of Life Living Food bars, which are loaded with probiotics, into their lunch bags.

healthy digestion and can be used during antibiotic therapy when most other probiotics are only recommended after antibiotic use.

One of the signs of poor digestive health is diarrhea, which health care professionals define as three or more loose, watery bowel movements per day. If your infant or toddler has the runs, then consider giving him or her a probiotic with *S. boulardii.* This live microorganism will help destroy pathogenic—or bad—bacteria in the bowels of your hurting youngster.

Infant diarrhea is a serious affliction in this country and one of the leading causes of childhood mortality outside our borders. (More than three million children die each year from diarrhea, mainly in underdeveloped countries, as compared to around five hundred a year in the United States.[10]) The central concern with infant diarrhea is that babies become dehydrated from the loss of body fluids.

Pediatricians often prescribe antibiotics for children with ear or respiratory tract infections, but antibiotics are a leading cause of diarrhea since they can destroy healthy bacteria that kids' young bodies need. To me, this underscores the importance of adding probiotics to their diets when diarrhea strikes or, even better, before it does. If symptoms persist for several days, however, be sure to see a pediatrician.

Since it's hard to find nutritional supplement companies that produce effective probiotic organisms suitable for children's digestive systems, I formulated a probiotic product called Primal Defense Kids. This probiotic supplement, which comes in a delicious banana flavor that youngsters love, supports healthy digestion and elimination and promotes a healthy immune response. Garden of Life also offers a delicious and convenient probiotic for older children and adults called Pro2Go, which is a delicious berry-flavored probiotic powder in single-serving sachets that resemble pixie sticks.

Don't Swing at This Pitch

Have you noticed the ads for a Diet Coke Plus, which is "fortified" with vitamins and minerals? How about the "enhanced" line of carbonated drinks from Pepsi, called Tava, that come with vitamins B, C, E, and chromium—the latter a nutrient tied to weight loss?

Sorry, but spiking soft drinks with synthetic minerals and vitamins to make them healthy is like adding rouge and eye shadow to a pig's face; it's still an ugly combination.

Some Whole Thoughts

At the beginning of this chapter, I mentioned that your children would be better off taking supplements produced from "whole food" sources. What do I mean by that?

Whole food supplements, by definition, are made from foods such as cereal grasses, broccoli, cauliflower, carrots, and berries. During the manufacturing process, these whole foods are compressed into a tablet or powdered form. Whole food supplements are closer to nature and much better for your children—and you—than vitamins formulated from nutrients that have been chemically isolated in the lab. Whole food nutritionals, also known as "living" vitamins and minerals in vitamin shops and health food stores, do not contain synthetic vitamins and minerals.

One of the most common supplements sold today is vitamin C, a go-to nutritional when Johnny comes home with the sniffles. A whole food version of vitamin C is a blend of acerola cherries, Indian gooseberries, oranges, grapefruits, and limes, along with juices pressed from red grapes, raspberries, blueberries, and strawberries. Important vitamins, minerals, and enzymes are extracted from the fruit, pulp, peel, and seeds, which makes whole food vitamin C more "bioavailable" to the body.

"Regular" vitamin C supplements found in supermarkets and pharmacies, however, list ascorbic acid as the first ingredient, but ascorbic acid is an isolated chemical that is only part of the vitamin C complex and *not* what

Thumbs Down on Vitamin Megadoses

There was a time, back in the 1970s and 1980s, when it was the fashion to take megadoses of vitamin C—up to 10,000 milligrams a day—to fight off a cold or flu. An influential book at that time was *Vitamin C and the Common Cold* by Linus Pauling, Ph.D., which encouraged folks to gulp down vitamin C tablets like M&Ms.

I'm not in favor of children *or* adults megadosing on vitamin C (or any other vitamins), however, because our bodies were not designed to consume these nutritionals in massive amounts. A common side effect of vitamin C megadoses is diarrhea, which is even more harmful to young children than adults. Taking ten 1,000-milligram tablets of vitamin C would give your youngster quite a colon cleanse, if you catch my drift, because that much vitamin C is like eating 150 oranges in a single day.

Not a healthy way to get your vitamin C.

you'd find in an orange. In addition, you can find some rather unnatural-sounding names printed on the ingredient list affixed to the back of the bottle or plastic container of vitamin C: croscarmellose, vegetable magnesium stearate, silica, vegetable stearic acid, cornstarch, cellulose gel, hydroxypropyl cellulose, hydroxypropyl methylcellulose, and polyethylene glycol. So which supplements sound like they come from natural sources and which ones were formulated in a researcher's laboratory?

When Johnny Comes Marching Home—with a Cold

If Johnny brings home the sniffles from preschool, I highly recommend going the homeopathic medicine route. Nicki and I have become great believers in homeopathic medicine as a safe and effective treatment for Joshua, and we keep a homeopathic first aid kit in the house if anything goes wrong. We've used C+ Cold Tablets from Highlands Homeopathic whenever Joshua starts coughing and sniffling.

Homeopathy is a system of medicine that treats illnesses by stimulating the body's own healing mechanisms. According to the *Encyclopedia of Natural Healing,* the foundation of homeopathy is that the body has an amazing ability to heal itself when the body's resistance to illness has weakened. Homeopathic remedies are natural and originate from plants, minerals, and animal sources. They work well for treatment of sore throats, stomachaches, and bouts of sneezing. This form of medicine, when used correctly, is ideal for all ages, especially infants and toddlers.

My experience with homeopathic medicine is that it's a very safe way to treat childhood colds and flu, and the good news is that you'll find out right away whether homeopathic medicine will help your son or daughter overcome some type of bug. The best way to introduce yourself to homeopathic medicine is drop by your local natural food store (Whole Foods, Wild Oats, or your independent health food store) and ask questions.

I recommend supplements that are from whole food sources and weren't synthetically created to imitate complex structures like vitamin C, vitamin E, or the B complex vitamins. Yes, synthetic versions of these vitamins are much more affordable: a warehouse club will let you cart off a five-hundred-pill bottle of 1,000-milligram vitamin C for less than ten bucks, while a whole food vitamin C will set you back twenty dollars for a bottle of ninety 500-milligram tablets. But like shopping for organic food, you get what you pay for when it comes to nutritional supplements. If you can afford the added expense, purchase your favorite vitamins and minerals from companies that manufacture whole food vitamins and minerals.

In closing, my philosophy is that even if children eat a lot of organic fruits and vegetables and consume whole grains and even cultured dairy products, they should still take a good omega-3 cod liver oil and a good children's probiotic supplement to provide nutrients that are critical to a child's growth.

R̶x THE GREAT PHYSICIAN'S Rx FOR CHILDREN'S HEALTH: SUPPLEMENT THEIR DIETS WITH WHOLE FOOD NUTRITIONAL SUPPLEMENTS

- *Add high omega-3 cod liver oil to your children's infant or toddler formula.*

- *If your children are older, look for ways to introduce high omega-3 cod liver oil into their diets, either through sipping spoonfuls, taking capsules, or adding it to certain foods.*

- *To promote digestion, elimination, and a healthy immune system, give your children probiotics.*

- *Learn the difference between whole food vitamins and those made from chemically isolated nutrients.*

- *Consider homeopathic medicines for dealing with colds and sniffles.*

Take Action

To learn how to incorporate the principals of supplementing your children's diets with whole food nutritionals, please turn to page 176 for the Great Physician's Rx for Children's Health Seven-Day Plan.

KEY #3

Introduce Your Children to Advanced Hygiene

Nicki and I are feeling pretty good about ourselves: we're the parents of a three-year-old son who's potty-trained.

Now, how we got there is a book in itself, but for the longest time, it seemed like Joshua would *never* learn one of the most fundamental behaviors of human nature. Joshua got the pee pee in the potty down rather quickly; it was the stinky in the potty that proved to be a problem.

Though it took a year of constant coaching, I'm proud to say we've successfully trained Joshua to cleanse his hands—and use soap—after a trip to the bathroom. Now I'm confident that when he is not under our supervision—like at preschool—he'll continue to wash his hands after using the lavatory. I wonder, though, if he'll be a minority in his class.

Why do I say that? It's my belief that too many young children aren't being successfully taught *the* single most important act of personal hygiene. They're not hearing the message that washing their hands at the appropriate times will lead to healthier lives and help them avoid picking up the "crud" going around school and bringing it home to infect others.

By teaching your children—and adopting yourself—the elements of a protocol that I call "advanced hygiene," your bodies will be protected from germs, viruses, and microbial agents that rob you of vitality and energy. Every bit as essential to good health as diet and exercise, advanced hygiene will greatly increase the odds of your children staying healthy, which means there's a stronger chance that *you* will remain healthy as well.

Fear Factor

I fly somewhere nearly every week of the year, and I'm amazed—and grossed out—by how many guys don't wash their hands after going to the bathroom. They do their thing at the urinal, zip up, and depart the crowded restroom without so much as a glance at the washbasins. Why are men so lame about the most basic ingredient of good hygiene—washing their hands after they urinate?

Many feel that if they don't get pee on their hands, they've earned a free pass. Others believe that "clean freaks" like me are overreacting. I think there's another category at work here: some guys actually couldn't care less about washing their hands and practicing good hygiene.

Nicki says she's also grossed out whenever someone—usually a young thing in her teens or early twenties—leaves the toilet stall without washing her hands. If she does stop by the washbasin, she says, the young lady runs a brush through her hair or touches up her makeup with unwashed hands. Let's just say she doesn't leave the restroom smelling like a rose.

Polling organizations and research groups over the years have surreptitiously monitored who's washing and who isn't. Generally speaking, around one-fourth of the population doesn't trouble themselves to wash up, with guys faring worse than the fairer sex, as just about anyone would predict. One of the latest observational surveys, conducted by the Harris Interactive research group in 2005, stationed monitors in public restrooms at airports and ballparks around the country. The results: 82 percent overall washed their hands after using the facilities. Women, as expected, were hands-down better than the men: 90 percent of women washed their hands, compared with only 75 percent of the men.[1]

I'm always dumbfounded when I witness this type of nasty behavior. Then again, men's restrooms at airports, stadiums, public parks, and gas stations have to be the most yucky places on the planet. It's so bad that if they told guys to aim for the floor, they might hit the urinals. It's just disgusting beyond belief. After I finish washing my hands, I practically do a combination of Tae Kwon Do and disco dancing to get out of there. I use my elbow to push on the door latch and jam my knee between the door and the doorjamb.

Whatever.

There's not a square inch of sanitary cleanliness in these public restrooms, which is why I wonder what the mother of a three-year-old was thinking when she escorted her *barefoot* son into the women's restroom at Atlanta's Hartsfield Airport! (I also question if celebrity Britney Spears lost her thinking cap when she was photographed leaving a Santa Barbara gas station restroom clad in bare feet. Talk about nasty! "It remains to be hoped that she at least washed her hands," opined one blogger.[2])

Listen, I'm not obsessive-compulsive about hygiene like Howard Hughes, the 1930s aviator who washed his hands until they bled raw. Nor am I similar to another Howard—Howie Mandel, host of the popular NBC game show *Deal or No Deal,* who won't shake hands with contestants. He'll hug or bump knuckles, but Howie won't press the flesh because he doesn't want to pick up their germs.[3] At least he can joke about it: when asked by *Sports Illustrated* if he could trade places with an athlete for a day, who would it be, Mandel quipped, "I'm such a germaphobe, I don't want to be in anyone's shoes besides my own."[4]

That line is probably part of Howie Mandel's stand-up act in Las Vegas, but I understand where he's coming from, especially with the hand-shaking thing. The greatest opportunity for germs to infect another person is when we grip another person's hand in ours. When that moment of touch occurs, tiny microbes are passed from one individual to another—microbes that have been hanging out in the soft tissues underneath our fingernails. The exchange happens because germs are more easily spread by hand-to-hand contact than airborne exposure—like when somebody sneezes in your vicinity. "Germs don't fly; they hitchhike," declared Australian scientist Kenneth Seaton, Ph.D., who made it his life's work to convince the medical establishment that hand-to-hand transmission is the most efficient mechanism for spreading germs.

So if somebody shakes your hand . . . someone who didn't wash up after going to the bathroom or changing a dirty diaper, then you're quite vulnerable to picking up *their* germs on *your* fingertips. Once these nomadic bacteria pitch camp in the soft tissues around and under your fingernail, it's a matter of time before you rub your eyes, scratch your nose, stroke your ears, or touch your mouth. When any of those instinctive behaviors occur, the transfer of germs has been set into motion. Soon—very soon—your body's immune system will come under a blistering attack as the germs, moving relentlessly like Roman foot soldiers, invade the portals to your body. Before you can say, "I think I'm coming down with something," you're reaching for a tissue to dry your runny nose or catch a rip-roaring sneeze.

Maybe you haven't paid attention to how easily germs enter the body through the nasal passageway or the corner of the eyes—the tear ducts—when you touch those areas. All of us involuntarily rub our faces so often that we don't even know we're doing it half the time, but when skin-on-skin or skin-on-membrane contact is made, you transfer a garden variety of bacteria, allergens, environmental toxins, and viruses from one part of the body to another. In medical terms, it's called auto- or self-inoculation of the conjunctival (eyes) or nasal (nose) mucosa with a contaminated finger.

Classroom Test

Dr. Kenneth Seaton, a research scientist, once commenced a study in which ten healthy people were put into a room with ten other people suffering an active virus. They spent eight hours in close proximity but were not allowed any physical contact. At the end of the day, tests were conducted. Only two of the ten people picked up the bug.

Dr. Seaton repeated the same experiment with ten sick people and ten healthy folks, but this time he allowed and even encouraged physical contact. After eight hours of high fives, low fives, and handshakes in between, you can predict what happened next: all ten healthy people got sick.

Sharing this scientific knowledge with your young children will pass right over their cute heads, but I wanted to relay this important information so that you will have a concrete understanding of the science of good hygiene and the tools to protect your children from picking up germs—germs that can be passed on to you. Let's face it: we touch our children *a lot* throughout the course of a day. We're constantly stroking a child's hands and fingers, cleaning up their drool, touching their faces, and changing dirty diapers—everyday activities that raise the opportunity for child-to-parent transmission of germs and viruses, as any parent who's ever picked up a flu "that's going around" will attest.

If your children attend a day care, preschool, or elementary school, I'll guarantee you that they're exposed to germs on doorknobs, computer mouses, playground equipment, carpets, floors, toilets, and sinks every single day. When inquisitive children touch these contaminated surfaces, they're susceptible to infection—and bringing those germs home with them.

Beware of the Dreaded Shopping Cart

You and your little one waddle toward the entrance of your local supermarket, where you lift your fourteen-month-old son into the seat of a shopping cart. He naturally grabs the handlebar as you push the cart into the gleaming store—a bar that feels slimy to your touch. Every minute is a constant battle to stop your rambunctious son from putting one of his hands into his mouth—the hand that's been clutching the shopping cart handle.

And germs are dancing for joy.

Shopping carts are wonderful inventions, but they also happen to be incredibly dirty at the same time. Few mothers are aware that shopping carts are Traveling Bacteria Shows that carry 1.4 million bacteria per square inch, a thousand times more bacteria than found on a toilet seat.[5] The University of Arizona Environmental Research Laboratory discovered that 21 percent of shopping carts contain a potpourri of bodily fluids, including foul microbes like staphylococcus anureus, streptococcus pneumonia, E. coli, and hepatitis B.[6]

It's enough to make you want to carry a box of surgical gloves to the store, but that won't protect the precious children in your care unless you take steps to clean up the shopping cart. I recommend bringing along a box of disinfectant wipes when you go shopping and wipe off the shopping cart before depositing your child into his or her seat.

Thankfully, the message of dirty shopping carts is finding an audience. Supermarket chains like Publix, Kroger, and Andersons, along with progressive natural food markets like Whole Foods, are supplying disinfectant wipes that customers can grab to decontaminate their shopping carts to their heart's content. Another option would be purchasing products like a Buggy Bag or Shopper Topper that you can plop over the cart seat.

Better yet, I urge you to store a box of disinfectant wipes in the car or your purse. Disinfectant wipes from SaniCart or Clorox are part of a $1.5 billion business growing at a healthy 6 percent clip a year, and the Environmental Protection Agency has certified several wipes against certain flu bugs, food contaminants, and *Pseudomonas aeruginosa*, which is associated with infections of skin, respiratory, and gastrointestinal tracts.[7]

Since Nicki and I are well aware that Joshua could be bringing home microscopic hitchhikers from his preschool, as well as the church nursery, we're motivated to introduce our toddler-aged son to advanced hygiene. The first step is teaching him how to scrub his hands and fingers with a special semisoft hand soap that we keep by his bathroom sink. (You can visit www.BiblicalHealthInstitute.com and click on the Resource Guide for my recommendations on which semisoft soap to purchase.)

The creamy-type soap, which usually comes in a white tub and is rich in essential oils, removes germs from underneath the fingernails. We're tutoring Joshua to lather the soap over his cuticles and pay extra attention to areas under the fingernails, but he's been more interested in making a gooey mess than listening to us. That's okay. When he's older, we'll make sure he gives the cuticles and fingernails the attention they need.

As for myself, I not only like jabbing my fingers into the tub of semisoft soap in our master bathroom, but I *can't wait* to cleanse my hands when I'm on the road. Airline flights, especially during the flu-and-cold season, are nothing more than flying germ farms. It's no secret that many airlines, under pressure to cut costs, don't clean their planes as often as they used to. Delta Airlines, which is battling back from bankruptcy, used to "detail" their planes every thirty days or so, but the legacy carrier allowed their deep-cleaning schedules to lapse to every sixteen months as a cost-cutting measure.

I'm a Platinum Medallion frequent flier with Delta (I fly the airline often from West Palm Beach to the Atlanta hub and on to my final destination), so believe me, I noticed when the fleet became dingy and dirty. Gratefully, Delta has returned to its old deep-cleaning schedule, but I still wonder—no matter what airline I fly—what germs lurk on the armrests and tray tables, the toilet seats and handles, and the doorknobs coming in and out of the planes' bathrooms.

You Can't Beat Soap and Water
by Dr. Fiona Blair

I'm glad to hear that Jordan uses organic hand sanitizers, which are the next best thing when you can't get to a faucet to thoroughly wash your hands in semisoft soap. At the same time, I want to caution readers not to rely on hand sanitizers, many of which claim to kill 99.9 percent of bacteria.

I wonder what's lurking in that other .1 percent. What I mean is that a sanitizer is different from the disinfectants that doctors routinely use because disinfectants must completely eliminate all the organisms listed on its label. And one other thing about antimicrobial hand sanitizers: they're tested on inanimate objects, not human skin. They're proven to be no more effective than regular soap and water, just more expensive.

I still think that washing warm water over your hands, with soap, gets the job done better than hand sanitizers, but that's just a pediatrician speaking.

Once I'm on the ground, I retreat to the nearest bathroom and clean my hands with an organic hand sanitizer. Sometimes I wait until I reach my hotel, where I will dip my fingers into a tub of semisoft soap to rid myself of any germs I may have picked up on the plane. Then I rinse my hands thoroughly before heading off to a business appointment, speaking engagement, or book-signing event.

I speak at churches and conferences probably twenty weekends a year, but, unlike Howie Mandel, I don't mind shaking hands because I genuinely enjoy greeting people in this manner. At the same time, however, I'm well aware that my hands are picking up microbial hitchhikers from the dozens, if not hundreds, of people who grip my right hand that day. When I return to my hotel room, the first thing I do is wash my hands with my special semisoft soap, rinsing them with running water as warm as I can stand.

Cleaning Up after Cleaning Him Up

While I'm concerned with what's on my hands after I shake hands at a book signing, I would imagine that parents are more concerned with cleaning their hands after changing a dirty diaper.

When shopping for wipes to use when changing diapers, I prefer natural ones that aren't as harsh to the skin as commercial wipes, many of which contain harmful phenols, aldehydes, or alcohol. If you use these commercial wipes to clean up your children's bottoms, you'll wipe natural oils off their skin—oils effective in fighting off germs—and introduce potential toxins to their bodies.

I recommend baby wipes from a company called Seventh Generation, which produces unscented wipes that haven't been bleached with chlorine and do not contain alcohol or synthetic ingredients that can irritate a baby's skin.

How long and how thoroughly should you wash your hands? An Australian observational study of two hundred people washing their hands at public toilets revealed that only 7 percent of males and 20 percent of females washed their hands for at least ten seconds and rinsed and dried for at least ten seconds.[8]

The Australians have as much to learn about good hygiene as Americans. Washing your hands properly is a little more involved than just running warm water over your soapy hands. Here is a refresher course that you can follow:

1. Wet your hands with water as warm as you can stand.

2. Open the tub of semisoft soap and dig your fingernails into the soft cream. Add a dab to the palms of both hands.

3. Rub your hands vigorously. Work the soap into the soft tissues underneath your fingernails, where armies of germs and viruses lie in wait to attack.

4. Scrub for at least fifteen seconds—not ten seconds—while singing "Happy Birthday" all the way through.

5. Rinse well and dry your hands on a paper towel or clean cloth towel. When I'm in a public restroom, I'll use a paper towel to turn off the running water and open the exit door. Sometimes I've had to jam my foot in the door while I pretzel my body like a Cirque du Soleil performer in order to toss the paper towel into a nearby trash can, but I'll gladly torque my body rather than touch a dirty doorknob.

Share these principles with your children. Make hand washing fun, not a chore. Toddlers love "playing" with water, and they will gladly mimic what you do. If your children are in the primary school years, however, they might think it's too childish to sing "Happy Birthday" while washing up, so you might talk about how everyone gets "cooties" on their hands. The hygienic response, you say, would be cleaning those hands before you infect yourself—and others—with someone else's icky germs.

When it comes to your children, you know best how to get the main point across—that washing your hands after you go to the bathroom is imperative. I'll leave this how-to aspect of good parenting in your hands.

Clean hands, I hope.

I know that I've just made the simple task of hand washing sound involved, but there's more to advanced hygiene. The next step is dipping your face into a bathroom sink filled with a mineral-based water solution. This step of advanced hygiene is known as a *facial dip*, which I often call "sink snorkeling" when I speak in front of an audience.

A facial dip begins with filling a washbasin or clean, large bowl with warm but not hot water. Then I pour one to three tablespoons of table salt and two eyedroppers of an iodine-based mineral solution into the water. Next, I swirl the water with my hands. Then I bend over and dunk my face into the water, opening my eyes several times to allow the cleansing water to flush out the membranes around my eyes.

After performing this chore several times, I dunk my face one last time, but this time I keep my eyes closed and my mouth out of the water while I blow bubbles through my nose. This act allows the minerals in the water to "Roto-Rooter" my nasal membrane, clearing the nostrils of any germs residing there. If one of my nostrils is clogged up from the sniffles, I close the open nostril while underwater and slowly inhale to draw the diluted facial solution into the blocked nostril. That maneuver usually unplugs the nostril.

I execute these facial dips religiously morning and evening, but when I'm fighting a cold or flu, I'll perform the facial wash every few hours until I feel better. It's amazing how the flu and cold symptoms usually depart within twenty-four hours whenever I use this technique.

Facial dips are the "advanced" part of advanced hygiene, and I know that Joshua isn't quite mature enough to put this second step all together. He's seen Daddy and Mommy blow bubbles and has given it a go, but I would imagine that we're still a couple of years away from his totally getting how to close an open nostril and fill the plugged nostril with solution by drawing in a breath.

The last step of advanced hygiene involves dropping very diluted drops of hydrogen peroxide and minerals into the ears to cleanse the ear canal. Whenever we suspect Joshua has an earache or acts cranky, we introduce this cleansing solution into his ears. Nicki and I believe that this is a major reason why our son has avoided the dreaded ear infections common among infants and toddlers.

Like eating foods that God created and supplementing their diets with certain key nutritionals, advanced hygiene should become foundational in your children's lives. As they get older, remind them that the old Hebrew proverb, "Cleanliness is next to godliness," gained currency for a good reason.

Bath Time

Joshua is all boy when it comes to taking his daily bath. He loves splashing around in the water and making a mess, which makes him a perfectly normal kid.

Nicki and I have tried to make Joshua's daily bath much more than just a way to clean him up after another day of running around the house or exploring the backyard. We add an oil blend that includes peppermint oil and eucalyptus oil to Joshua's bath that he can breathe in to help his immune system. Whenever Nicki or I approach his bathtub holding a brown bottle filled with these essential oils, he calls them "raindrops." If Joshua shows signs of sniffling, we'll rub some of these "raindrops" on his chest or put a few drops on his pillow that he can inhale as he's falling asleep. Aubrey Organics, a company listed in the Resource Guide in the back of this book, sells a variety of bath oils you can try.

Let Them Eat Dirt

You might find this next statement off the wall after devoting most of this chapter to washing your hands, but whenever we can, we allow our son to play in the dirt.

Go ahead, Joshua. Get dirty.

We're encouraging him to dig his hands into backyard soil so that his immune system gets some practice fighting bacteria and viruses. In children's early years, their immune systems need to be stimulated by bacteria so that their immune systems can reach full strength. A growing number of scientists theorize that an immature immune system triggers a host of illnesses, including asthma, allergies, and autoimmune diseases like rheumatoid arthritis and severe forms of diabetes. This new train of thought is called the "hygiene hypothesis" by researchers, and it only underscores the importance of early childhood exposure to microbes. By exposing your children to natural germs today, I believe you are helping them develop strong immune systems for the future.

The "hygiene hypothesis," first put forward by British medical researcher David P. Strachan in 1989, states that our immune systems have two types of lymphocytes, or white blood cells, called Th1 and Th2 (kind of like the twin mischief-makers Thing One and Thing Two in Dr. Seuss's classic book *The Cat in the Hat*). Th1 lymphocytes respond primarily to bacteria and viruses, while Th2 lymphocytes respond primarily to parasites.

Usually, Th1 and Th2 lymphocytes balance each other out, but when your children's immune system isn't challenged by enough viruses and bacteria, they could wind up with an underdeveloped Th1 system or an overdeveloped Th2 system. Some researchers believe that the high incidence of asthma in inner-city children is directly related to the lack of dirt in that environment. The National Heart, Lung, and Blood Institute estimates that the incidence of asthma in children younger than four is nearly three times what it was in 1980.[9] And in Germany, the Association of German Allergists concluded a study showing that children who grew up on farms had fewer allergies than their counterparts in urban areas.[10]

Germs found naturally in the soil and plants are different from the germs your child would pick up from other children. The unfortunate reality is that germs passed from one human to another—through touching—are almost always human fecal germs. What we want to do is expose our son to germs outside in the environment, both good and bad, to help train his immune response. Dr. Strachan, as well as a growing number of medical researchers, believes that the microorganisms found in dirt influence the maturation of the immune system. The British epidemiologist says that older children who come home dirty are actually doing their younger siblings a favor because they're exposing their budding immune systems to microbes that cause them to build antibodies.

Since our family lives in suburbia, Nicki and I feel as though we are playing catch-up with getting Joshua outside more. For the first two and a half years of his life, we resided in a zero-lot-line neighborhood, which meant backyards the size of postage stamps; limited fencing; and narrow, five-foot setbacks between homes. After Joshua started walking, it wasn't prudent to let him run outside. I also noticed that the lawn service was constantly spraying the St. Augustine grass, a coarse turf surrounding each house, with herbicides and pesticides.

The lack of a suitable backyard is one of the reasons we moved to an established neighborhood with generous lot sizes when Joshua turned two and a half. Now our son has some room to roam inside our fenced backyard, and he likes sticking his fingers into the organic lettuce growing in my hydroponic tower garden. If he plays in the dirt, I don't mind him coming back to the house with grubby hands.

One play set you won't find in our new backyard is a sandbox. A sandbox isn't as healthy as playing in the dirt because dirt is a living ecosystem, while sand is not. Sand has a way of preserving germs left in the box—like the deposits from neighborhood cats that mistake the sandbox for a litter box.

When it comes to your children and your backyard, remember this:

- Dirt, yes.

- Grass, yes, unless it's been recently sprayed.

- Sandbox, no, unless it's covered when not in use.

So Clean You Could Eat Off The . . .

I was asked one time if I practice the "five-second rule," which means that if a piece of cheese or a cracker falls to the floor but is picked up within five seconds, it is still safe to eat.

My opinion is colored by a childhood memory of my younger sister, Jenna, finding a piece of gum on the floor of a K-Mart when she was three years old. As toddlers are wont to do, she stuck the gum in her mouth. Talk about how to get sick in a hurry! Jenna never pulled that stunt again.

I haven't witnessed Joshua picking up disgusting things off the floor and eating them. If that happened, though, I don't think it would be a problem in our house because Nicki is very neat and keeps the kitchen floor spotless. As for the five-second rule, I would say that depending on the food that hit the floor, he should be all right. A cracker with peanut butter seems to always land on the peanut-butter side, so that would be a no-no, but if a grape or blueberry fell to the floor, why not let him eat it? After rinsing the fruit under the kitchen faucet, of course.

As we just learned in the section about letting your kids play in the dirt, sometimes a few innocuous germs are good for your children's immune systems. We drew the line, though, when Joshua's pacifier hit the deck. Nicki or I rinsed his "passie" with hot water every time it popped out of his mouth.

Circumstantial Evidence

Not long after my wife, Nicki, and I learned that we would become proud parents of a baby boy—thanks to an ultrasound in her fifth month—we put that information to good use. We finished decorating his bedroom in accents of baby blue and informed the family so they could buy the right clothes for the baby.

When we heard that we would be bringing a son into this world, I also mentally prepared myself for Joshua's circumcision. The decision of whether to circumcise Joshua was a no-brainer for two reasons:

1. In Genesis 17:10–14, God directed Abraham to circumcise himself, his household, and his slaves as part of an everlasting covenant in which God promised to make Abraham the father of a multitude of nations.

2. I believe God's Word is always backed up by science, and if the Creator ordained circumcision on the eighth day of a boy's life, then I know He had His reasons.

We had Joshua circumcised in our home by a *mohel* (pronounced *moyle*), usually a Jewish rabbi or physician who performs the religious ceremony/medical procedure. The cutting away of his tiny foreskin wasn't easy to watch, but I felt great satisfaction knowing that I was fulfilling a directive from God and welcoming Joshua into a family that included Abraham, Isaac, Jacob, Moses, Joshua, David, and our Savior Jesus, as well as my male ancestors. Both of my parents are Jewish, but when I was born, Dad was in naturopathic school where he was taught that circumcision was a barbaric practice unnecessary in today's enlightened times. Fortunately, someone convinced him that I should be circumcised, and that happened when I was around three weeks old.

From what I hear, though, circumcision—whether performed as part of a *bris milah* ceremony or in a doctor's office—is on the wane these days. Since the early 1980s, hospital circumcision rates have fallen steadily as parents wonder whether they should allow their son's foreskin—the sensitive sleeve of skin covering the head of the penis—to be snipped away.

Back in the 1960s, circumcision rates were a sky-high 95 percent, but by 2004, that figure had dropped to around 57 percent,[11] and today, according to the National Center for Health Statistics, newborn circumcision rates vary by geographic region. Baby boys in the Midwest are circumcised more than anywhere else in the country, while out West, circumcision rates have fallen off a cliff: only 37 percent of boys undergo the procedure.[12] Demographers say the dramatic decline in states like California and Arizona reflects the increased birth rate among Hispanics, who are less likely to subject their infant sons to circumcision.

In all corners of the country, neonatal circumcision has become a controversial subject. A noisy group of circumcision protesters have picketed hospitals in recent years, carrying signs that read, "Peace begins with how we treat our children." Men claiming that they were sexually desensitized without their consent or that their parents were not fully informed before signing consent papers have filed lawsuits.

I'm afraid these well-meaning folks are misguided. As I said, God knew what He was doing when He introduced circumcision to His chosen people, although I would imagine that the idea of slicing off a part of your manhood sounded pretty far-out to Abraham, who was ninety-nine years old at the time. God required circumcision as a sign of obedience and as a visible sign that identified the male as a child of God forever. There was no way to reverse this procedure.

Some biblical scholars say that circumcision was a symbol of "cutting off" the old life of sin, but I believe God instituted the practice for health reasons as well; otherwise, why did He specifically say that newborn males must be circumcised on the eighth day of life? Modern medicine has discovered that the eighth day is an ideal time for a circumcision. Vitamin K, a necessary component for blood clotting, is normally at low levels in newborns, but this clotting agent rises *above* adult levels around the seventh day of life before settling in at adult levels around day ten. God had specific reasons for designating day eight as the best time to circumcise male newborns.

What also interests me is that modern medicine has established a link between circumcision and cancer. For instance, the overall rate of penile cancer in this country is low—about one case per one hundred thousand men—but when researchers studied eighty-nine men with invasive penile cancer, eighty-seven men, or 97 percent, had not been circumcised.[13]

In addition, women are less likely to develop cancer of the cervix if they are in a sexual relationship with a circumcised male rather than an uncircumcised male.[14] Circumcised men were half as likely to be infected with HPV, or human papilloma virus, a sexually transmitted disease.[15] HPV can cause cervical cancer.

If you're expecting a boy (or have a very young boy), I'm not suggesting that you look up *mohel* in the Yellow Pages and schedule a bris posthaste, but you should be aware that being uncircumcised puts him, as well as his future spouse, at greater risk for certain types of cancers.

Getting an Earful

The final section of advanced hygiene that I want to address is the ear infection, which is one of the most worrisome illnesses for children *and* parents to go through. You'll be interested in what my coauthor, Dr. Fiona Blair, has to say about ear infections from the viewpoint of a pediatrician who sees a *lot* of mothers bringing their crying children into her office, complaining of a major-league earache or tugging at their ears while acting irritable. Her comments can be found in the sidebar on page 103.

Pediatricians like Dr. Blair will tell you that ear infections come with the territory because children's immune systems don't fully develop until the age of seven, which means their little bodies have difficulties fighting infections. Children raised on formula, sent to day care at an early age, or exposed to cigarette smoke are more likely candidates for ear infections.[16]

I mentioned earlier that Joshua has avoided ear infections during the first three years of life. I credit this to a stellar diet brimming with extremely high nutrients, never missing a day of omega-3 cod liver oil, consuming probiotics, and living in a home with air purifiers. But I would also say that Joshua has been raised by parents who take advanced hygiene seriously, which could be a key explanation since physicians tell us most ear infections are caused by bacteria and viruses attacking the ear's eustachian tubes. I can tell you this: though a lot of my friends' kids get ear infections, *none* who have followed the Great Physician's prescription have rushed into a pediatrician's office seeking treatment for an ear infection.

At the same time, if your child has had an ear infection or two, that doesn't mean you are a bad parent or raising that little one in the wrong way. Stuff happens. Your toddler could complain that his ears are bothering him tomorrow, and if that happens, it may be because nasty bacteria and germs have successfully invaded his ear canal.

How would we treat our own son's ear infection? With all due respect to Dr. Blair, Nicki or I would first search for homeopathic answers before taking him to see our pediatrician. The conventional medicine approach—giving our son antibiotics—has been clearly overused, and these medicines can even be harmful.

So we'd rather take a proactive approach and teach Joshua the principles of advanced hygiene and continue to drip diluted drops of hydrogen peroxide and minerals into his ears. We're confident that cleansing his ear canals of bacteria and germs—and preventing those critters from reaching his fingertips—will protect him from experiencing a painful ear infection.

If your child comes down with a cold, a few drops of hydrogen peroxide into his ears could work wonders. I learned about this tip from Dr. Joe Mercola, but Dr. Blair tells me that when a child gets an ear infection, it occurs in the middle ear, behind the eardrum. "We know that membranes are permeable and that substances can cross them," she said. "Think about how your skin protects you from all the elements, but the skin can also absorb certain medications, so my theory is that the hydrogen peroxide crosses the eardrum and has an effect on the pathogens that may be in the middle ear."

According to the Mayo Clinic, children contract between six to ten upper respiratory illnesses a year—mostly during the cold-and-flu season between October and April. Keeping the ears clean can help tremendously. Back in 1928, Dr. Richard Simmons—not the fitness guru . . . he's not that old—hypothesized that cold and flu germs can sneak into the body through the ear canal. When you administer a few drops of hydrogen peroxide into each infected ear, your child may experience some bubbling or mild stinging, but the hydrogen peroxide seems to loosen up ears packed with wax and kill bacteria and viruses.

To be forewarned is to be forearmed. To help your children stave off viruses and bacteria, particular attention must be paid to practicing advanced hygiene because colds and flu are gifts that keep on giving—and parents always seem to be on the receiving end.

A Pediatrician's View of Ear Infections
by Dr. Fiona Blair

Next to the common cold, ear infections are among the most common diseases seen in pediatric practice: three out of four children suffer at least one infection by the time they reach three years of age. Ear infections—also called *acute otitis media*, or AOM—are more common in boys than girls.

Children, who often develop ear infections between the ages of two and four, do so because their Eustachian tubes are shorter and more horizontal than those of adults, which allows bacteria and viruses to find their way into the middle ear more easily. (The Eustachian tubes "pop" when you yawn or swallow as a plane begins its final descent.)

The pediatricians' playbook is uniformly standard: handing the mother a prescription for Amoxicillin or Augmentin—antibiotics commonly found to be effective for middle ear infections. The Mayo Clinic says that 50 percent of the antibiotics prescribed for preschoolers are used to treat ear infections. Researchers from Turku University Hospital in Finland identified a confection of pathogens that cause the great majority of ear infections in children. In 92 percent of the cases, bacteria caused the ear infection, followed by viruses in 70 percent of the cases.[17]

We know that ear infections caused by bacteria can spontaneously resolve themselves, and those caused by viruses do not respond to antibiotics. That's why in Europe pediatricians tend to adopt a wait-and-see approach to ear infections. After diagnosing an ear infection, they will tell the mothers to give their hurting child a pain reliever like Tylenol and watch him or her closely over the next twenty-four to forty-eight hours. If the child worsens in that time period, they are told to bring the child back to the pediatrician, at which time an antibiotic will be prescribed.

In this country, increasing rates of bacterial resistance to antibiotic treatment have raised concerns among pediatricians, and we've had discussions whether to adopt the wait-and-see European approach. That hasn't happened, however, and one of the major reasons is the fear of lawsuits. In rare instances, an ear infection can spread to the surrounding bone and cause a serious infection or even spread to the brain, resulting in meningitis.

Although very infrequent, the possibility of either of these events sends shivers down pediatricians' spines. In addition, we tend to want results quickly in this country, and the idea of waiting forty-eight hours for a resolution to a child's ear infection is not attractive to parents, so they demand an antibiotic.

This form of defensive medicine is why prescribing antibiotics is the standard treatment for a child's ear infection. Many natural health advocates such as Jordan believe that the overuse of antibiotics in children may set the stage for a lifetime of poor health, including allergies, fungal infections, and immune system disorders. The bottom line here is that antibiotics should be a treatment of last resort, not first choice.

R℞ THE GREAT PHYSICIAN'S Rx FOR CHILDREN'S HEALTH: INTRODUCE YOUR CHILDREN TO ADVANCED HYGIENE

- *Teach your children to wash up after every time they go to the bathroom. Then explain why they should clean their hands. Remind them that germs lurk everywhere, including doorknobs, computer keyboards at school, and classroom surfaces.*

- Purchase a semisoft soap with essential oils. Show your children how to dig their fingernails into the semisoft soap and work it into their cuticles and underneath their fingernails, where viruses and bacteria reside.

- When the children are older, show them how to perform a facial dip, which cleans the mucous membranes of their eyes as well as their nasal passageways.

- If you are expecting and know that you're having a boy, thoroughly consider circumcising your son.

- Cleanse their ear canals several times a week with very diluted drops of hydrogen peroxide and minerals, especially during the cold-and-flu season.

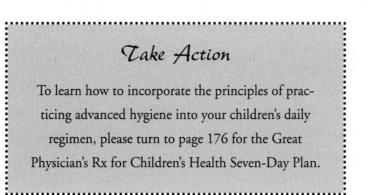

Take Action

To learn how to incorporate the principles of practicing advanced hygiene into your children's daily regimen, please turn to page 176 for the Great Physician's Rx for Children's Health Seven-Day Plan.

KEY #4

Condition Their Bodies with Exercise and Body Therapies

Nearly a century later, we can say the King of Sweden got caught up in the moment when handing Jim Thorpe his gold medals at the 1912 Olympic Summer Games, but I'm getting ahead of the story.

Jim Thorpe was born in Indian Territory in 1887—land now part of Oklahoma. The product of an Irish father and Sac and Fox Indian mother, he would be classified demographically as a Native American in today's times. His athletic career began in his teen years at Carlisle Indian Industrial School in Carlisle, Pennsylvania, where he was a natural in track and field as well as a star performer in football, baseball, lacrosse, and even ballroom dancing.

Jim was a marvel on the gridiron, a running back who swiveled his hips and left tacklers grasping at air. Future US president Dwight Eisenhower tried to bring down the swift Thorpe one time, but all he came up with for his effort was an injured knee. Years later, President Eisenhower said, "My memory goes back to Jim Thorpe. He never practiced in his life, and he could do anything better than any other football player I ever saw."[1]

I guess President Eisenhower never witnessed LaDanian Tomlinson shooting through a gap in the defensive line, but I digress. Although football was Jim Thorpe's favorite sport, track and field is where he would gain the most fame. At the 1912 Summer Olympics in Stockholm, Sweden, the American easily swept the competition in the decathlon and pentathlon. In those days, gold, silver, and bronze medals were presented to the top three finishers during the closing ceremonies of the Games. Legend has it that King Gustav of Sweden, when awarding Thorpe his gold medals, said, "You, sir, are the greatest athlete in the world," to which the modest American replied, "Thanks, King."

There's another legend surrounding Jim Thorpe, and it's that the "world's greatest athlete" was challenged—probably for money—to mimic everything a two-year-old boy did in a day—all the steps, all the running, all the jumping, all the energy. As you would expect, the supremely fit Thorpe ran out of gas in less than an hour. He couldn't keep up with an active toddler constantly on the move.

Any parent of an energetic toddler would confirm that even an athlete in as good shape as Jim Thorpe couldn't duplicate what a two-year-old rascal does in a day. Toddlers, by nature, have boundless reservoirs of energy and burn calories by the bushel. Their inquisitive personalities keep them on the move as they constantly explore their environments.

But something happens when the bambinos get older . . . they stop moving. They become capable of occupying themselves, playing quietly with Legos, Lincoln Logs, or Barbie dolls. They plop themselves in front of fifty-inch flat-screen TVs, where their eyeballs become glued to mesmerizing cartoon shows, Disney DVDs, wildlife documentaries on the Discovery Channel, and the latest PlayStation game. When children enter the tween years, computers vie for their attention—and often win. They can play *Grand Theft Auto* for hours on end, exercising only their thumbs and never realizing that their health is being carjacked.

While you can usually blame Happy Meal diets for tubby toddlers and portly preschoolers, when school-age lads and lasses pack on the pounds, you can also point the finger toward a cessation of physical activity. Experts agree that when it comes to childhood obesity, a diet of junk food and passive physical activity are the twin reasons why we're seeing ballooned waistlines and poor fitness among our youngsters. Fewer than 25 percent of children get any type of daily exercise.[2]

At a time when children should be at their physical peaks—running like the wind and jumping like jacks—their engines are idling. You can get them motoring on the right road by conditioning their bodies with exercise, making sure they get enough sleep and sunlight, and introducing them to hydrotherapy and music therapy, the fourth key that will unlock their health potential.

Junior Couch Potatoes in Training

It's not easy being a kid these days. The lure of five hundred cable channels, countless video games, burgers and fries, and sugary treats contribute to poor health, but several major studies, including one by the Centers for Disease Control and Prevention, have also linked suburban sprawl to childhood obesity. A national survey by researchers at Rutgers and Cornell revealed that 71 percent of adults said they walked or rode a bike to school when they were children, but only 22 percent walk or bike to school today. To paraphrase Winston Churchill, the rotund British statesmen, we shape our cities and then they shape us.[3]

Although I didn't hike six miles across frozen tundra to reach school, like my parents (ha!), I was one of those kids who pedaled his bike to high school. I don't see that happening with Joshua. We live in a fast-paced suburban setting, where the palm-lined thoroughfares are too dangerous to allow young children to ride their bikes *or* walk to school.

I'm sure Nicki will be chauffeuring our son everywhere. Like zillions of cul-de-sac suburbs across the fruited plain, Palm Beach Gardens is not pedestrian- or bike-friendly. The distances between our neighborhood and his school and soccer field will surely be problematic. Packed SUVs and bulky trucks zip along our six-lane boulevards at a fifty- or sixty-mile-per-hour clip, so it would be too dangerous to send a pint-sized boy out there and hope for the best.

If you live in a suburban neighborhood like ours, you're probably racking up the miles as you drive your kids everywhere—while they sit in the back watching *Cars* or *Finding Nemo* for the fiftieth time on the DVD player. So when do children get to exercise their limbs and lungs?

That's a question being asked a lot these days. If you're thinking that your kids will get a workout during recess, think again. School districts around the country, under pressure to "leave no child behind" and raise mandatory test scores, are shedding afternoon and sometimes morning recess to add more time in the classroom. The percentage of schools that don't have *any* recess ranges from 7 percent for first and second grades to 13 percent by sixth grade, according to government studies.[4]

I'm no child development expert, but common sense tells me that young students need a chance to blow off some steam. The notion that keeping children's bottoms glued to their chairs while cramming more teaching down their throats—with no breaks for physical activity or relaxation—flies in the face of rational thought. I don't see how you can keep a kid on task all day, especially since I was one of those live wires who couldn't wait for the recess bell to ring.

Give Me a Break

I'm also incensed about how elementary schools in Massachusetts, South Carolina, Wyoming, Washington, Oregon, and California have banned "chase" and "contact" games—like tag and dodgeball—on the pretext that children's tender psyches could be bruised. Administrators are also concerned about liability for injuries from touch football or soccer.

This is yet another example of coddling our youngsters and not looking at the greater good: frenetic exercise is essential to young, growing bodies, and there are life lessons to be learned from schoolyard competition, win or lose.

Dr. Joe Mercola says the elimination of free play at school recess is a shocking reflection on the state of US education. "Eliminating recess will only accelerate the epidemic of childhood obesity," he said. "It is nearly incomprehensible to me that school districts should ban one of the few activities left that promote health at school—playing independently at recess."[5]

Nicki and I haven't decided where Joshua will attend elementary school—we hope to put him in a Christian setting—but we won't enroll him where recess has been purged from the daily schedule. Children who run around the schoolyard not only keep their weight under control, but also perform better academically since their brains are receiving more blood. Olga Jarrett, a professor of early child education at Georgia State University, said her classroom studies show that children, when deprived of recess, cannot concentrate. They also lose focus and distract others.[6]

As for organized exercise, nearly a third of US states do not mandate physical education classes for elementary and middle school students, either. Almost one-fourth of states allow PE credits to be earned through online physical education courses.[7]

Online gym classes for kids.

Yeah, right. Somehow, I don't see that working.

Playtime

Whether or not your children's elementary or middle school offers recess and gym classes, this is not the time to sit on your duff. Your kids need to get moving, so what are your options for boosting their physical activity?

Of course, much depends on their age and maturity. Toddlers, as I said, run around the house like Tasmanian devils, so the last thing parents should do is let them watch Bugs Bunny outwit the Tasmanian Devil on Cartoon Network all afternoon. Although we are not averse to letting Joshua view a Disney DVD before bedtime, we monitor the TV closely, especially during the "dead time," late-afternoon hours. As long as he's running around the house or playing in the backyard, that's fine with us.

Preschoolers, kindergarteners, and first graders need unstructured time to play and unconstrained space to allow their imaginations to take flight. They should learn to exercise through everyday activities, like swinging on monkey bars and chasing their friends. They also need other children to play with. If yours is an only child, try to schedule opportunities for him or her to interact with your friends' children. Sometimes that's easier said than done, but it will be well worth the effort.

As your child gets older, consider enrolling him in gymnastic and exercise classes for children. You should check out what's offered at YMCAs, fitness centers, and private gyms and studios. Some gyms, like Fitwize 4 Kids, offer classes for moms *and* their toddlers/preschoolers. The instructors focus on making exercise fun.

For older kids, some fitness centers have adapted with the times by offering Dance Dance Revolution (DDR), a video game that requires players to follow the on-screen action with dance steps on a pressure-sensitive mat. Arrows scroll up the television screen to the beat of a song chosen by the player. As an arrow moves across the screen, the player steps on the corresponding arrow on the platform. Dance Dance Revolution is more difficult than it sounds and keeps kids moving.

I don't see Dance Dance Revolution in Joshua's future, but never say "never," right? When our son gets older, we'll introduce him to several sports—baseball, basketball, football, and soccer. (I especially love baseball, America's Pastime, and Joshua and I are into baseball memorabilia.) The ages of seven to eleven are when children become aware of their bodies and develop an interest in competition.

The elementary school years are the golden years for organized youth sports, and in the States these days, that usually means soccer. Estimates of how many children play soccer are hard to come by since there's no database of soccer organizations, but all I know is that every time I pass a park on Saturday morning, I see a scrum of kids chasing a black-and-white ball like bumblebees. I can understand why millions of preadolescent children are involved in soccer because it's a simple game—run and kick a ball toward a goal. Soccer demands lung-bursting running that's great for kids' cardiovascular systems and burning up calories.

The primary school years are also a good time to introduce youngsters to a great exercise program known as *functional fitness*. If you're scratching your head, functional fitness is a series of full-body movements that work major muscle groups in their full range of motion. Functional training is great for all ages—from seven to ninety-seven years old—and increases athletic ability, speed, agility, and balance.

In my early twenties, I was a personal trainer who taught classes in functional fitness, which is known in some fitness clubs as *purposeful training*. During that time, I learned that adults and children look at exercise differently. Physically mature men and women exercise to improve their health, lose a few pounds, and better their appearance, but children aren't interested in those things. Kids exercise to have fun, make friends, and learn something new, so taking six-year-old Junior to your neighborhood fitness center and plopping him on an elliptical trainer borders on the ridiculous.

I didn't train many children under the age of twelve, but when parents did sign up their youngsters, my goal was to improve their cardiovascular fitness, overall flexibility, and motor skills by having them complete a half hour or hour of functional fitness exercises with me. Performing squats, upper-body "lifts" with simple household items like water bottles or cans of tomato sauce, or overhead "presses" helped their growing bodies stay agile, flexible, and resistant. I kept the functional fitness fast-paced and constantly changing to hold their attention.

I'm enjoying "working out" with Joshua in our home gym. I encourage him to jump on the trampoline, hang from the pull-up and dip station, and do squats with his very own two-pound dumbbells.

At Least It's a Start

I'm happy to learn that nonprofit organizations like Functional Fitness 4 Kids (FF4K) are offering free functional fitness classes for fourth through eighth graders. Children participate in after-school workouts designed to decrease body fat and increase strength and endurance. The program is currently offered in the northern Virginia/Washington, D.C. area with a goal of expanding the concept nationwide.

My favorite functional fitness exercises for kids revolve around simple exercises that you can do in the living room with your children. The first functional fitness movement you can lead them through is an *alternate overhead press*. Begin by standing with your feet shoulder-width apart. Tell your children to keep their tummies straight. Then fully extend your right arm, with the palm facing up, telling your kids it's like pretending to push a box skyward. As your right arm comes down, make the same motion with the left arm, palm up. Start with five repetitions with each arm, building up to ten or twenty.

You can make the alternate overhead press more fun by letting the kids choose a small can of vegetables from the pantry. Lifting the can into the air provides enough resistance to build their arm and shoulder muscles.

The second exercise you can show your kids is a *bicep curl*. It's an easy one as well. Take both arms and stretch them out at your thighs with both hands facing down. Have them curl each arm, one at a time, bending only at the elbow. Start with five curls; then go to ten. A more advanced position would be pulling one elbow up to shoulder height and making a motion similar to pulling a lawn mower starting cord.

Squats aren't easy for adults, but kids are so limber that they can do them by the dozen. Teach them how to do a proper squat, though. Begin with the feet shoulder-width apart. Squat down as far as you comfortably can with your arms stretched out for balance and your palms facing down. Dip toward the ground. After twenty squats, you'll be feeling the burn, but your kids will be ready for more.

Lunges are another functional exercise where technique is important. Show your kids how to bend their backs and touch their toes while they lunge forward with one large step. This functional lunge will aid in the strength of their legs and glutes as well as improve flexibility in their backs.

You might consider taking several functional fitness classes before trying these with your children. Many of the national chains—Gold's Gym, LA

Functional Fitness at Bedtime

This is either a great idea or a lousy one, but I think a good time to lead your children in functional fitness is just before bedtime. As any experienced parent will attest, kids will do almost anything to delay going to bed, so they'll be eager to exercise with you. Since you'll also get some exercise from leading them through the functional fitness movements, there are benefits on both sides.

The problem is that elevating their heartbeats will wind them up, making it more difficult to put them down, but I think it's worth a try, especially if you choose the less energetic functional fitness exercises.

Fitness, Bally Total Fitness, as well as local YMCAs—offer classes in functional fitness. Good instructors can explain how to perform these movements properly, which will help you when you lead your youngsters in some physical activity. You'll also discover *why* functional fitness is so beneficial to the body. (For more information on functional fitness, along with a variety of different exercises, visit www.BiblicalHealthInstitute.com.)

Finally, I recommend that you invest in a mini-trampoline because jumping is one of the best lung-bursting exercises out there for kids. I've yet to meet any youngsters who don't naturally enjoy jumping up and down, up and down, up and down, because at the top of their bounce, their little bodies are in a state of weightlessness. Each deep bounce at the bottom of a jump subjects kids to two to three times the force of gravity, while at the top of the bounce, they experience the light-headed feeling of zero gravitational pull. For a split-second, they're floating above the world!

A mini-trampoline, also known as a rebounder, is typically three feet in diameter and about nine inches high, so they're safe—unless you let your children jump above a tiled or stone floor, of course. (Indoor rebounders are much safer than full-sized outdoor trampolines, which are higher off the ground and have a reputation for breaking a few arms—and necks—over the years.)

Jumping on a mini-trampoline does a lot more than let your kids burn off their afternoon snack, though. Rebounders are actually one of the best and most complete exercises they can do since jumping strengthens muscles, tendons, and ligaments. The acceleration, deceleration, and gravity pull positively stresses their young bones, which results in higher bone density. Rebounding affects every organ of their growing bodies and is directly related to the efficiency of the lymphatic system, which produces and stores cells that fight infection.

Many people are not aware that the lymphatic system, unlike the body's cardiovascular system that uses the heart to pump blood and oxygen cells through the veins and arteries, has no pump. The lymphatic system relies on body movement to open and close the one-way valves that transport lymphatic cells throughout the body and release toxic buildup. The up-and-down rhythmic bouncing causes all of the lymphatic system's one-way valves to open up, which increases flow by as much as fifteen times. Instead of germs, viruses, and bacteria remaining locked within the lymphatic system, jumping around on a rebounder breaks up the inertia and sends the germs and toxins on their way to elimination by the body.

Lymphologist C. Samuel West, N.D., author of *The Golden Seven Plus One*, said, "The tissues of the body, which comprise bones, flesh, and organs, excrete waste products as a result of their daily work. These must be quickly removed, or the tissues involved will suffer damage."[8] For adults, this damage could mean degenerative disease as well as an increase in the rate of aging.

That's why children—it's important to start young—need movement, muscular stimulation, and impact exercises like jumping. Whenever I have caught Joshua jumping on his bed, I couldn't bring myself to scold him because his rambunctious behavior was physically good for him. I had read about Dr. West's work and learned that when the lymphatic system is not stimulated from weight-bearing exercise, the cells become deprived of oxygen, which affects the body's ability to get rid of waste material. While the cardiovascular system circulates life-giving nutrients, the lymphatic system is more like a garbage collector that picks up toxins and metabolic junk from the cellular fluid of every organ. Jumping on a mini-trampoline is one way to get the garbage truck out of the garage and on the way to the dump.

Leaping on a mini-trampoline pairs wonderfully with functional fitness. You can have your child jump on the rebounder for two or three minutes while you perform some of the aforementioned full-body movements, and then switch places: you jump while he or she performs overhead presses or bicep curls. Your children will probably laugh as Mommy or Daddy jumps high in the air because for a split-second, you are out of control at the top of your bounce—and it shows! Five or ten minutes of functional fitness and rebounding is a great place to start down the road toward family fitness, and you can get your bodies moving any time of day.

Mini-trampolines are available at large merchandise and sporting goods stores. You can find good ones for less than fifty dollars, and many come with videos that you can follow as you or your child jump away.

So don't forget: youngsters love to jump for joy. Turn that enjoyment into even better health.

Bone Up on Exercise
By Dr. Fiona Blair

We've talked about the importance of diet and nutritional supplements for growing strong bones, but exercise has the greatest effect on bone mineral density during childhood and puberty. Just as muscles get stronger through use, the same principle applies to bones: the more work they do, the stronger they get.

The best exercises to build strong bones are weight-bearing activities: walking, running, hiking, skateboarding, dancing, basketball, tennis, gymnastics, volleyball, and soccer. I'm also a fan of jumping on mini-trampolines, as Jordan talks about. Swimming and biking, though superb cardiovascular pursuits, don't build bone density because they aren't weight-bearing exercises.

When children grow out of infancy, they need to move around! From my vantage point, too many young children aren't physically active these days. They're becoming "screen potatoes" because they sit in front of a TV or computer screen, playing video games instead of getting outside and playing with their friends.

Children, like river streams and commuter traffic, will take the path of least resistance. If you let them watch TV or play *Madden NFL* video games from the moment they get home from school until dinnertime, they'll gravitate toward those activities because they involve no physical effort. They'll sit there like bumps on a log, passive and unresponsive.

Instead, look for ways to get them moving and using those growing muscles.

Lullaby Time

It's one of the most overused sayings in the English language: *I slept like a baby last night.*

Whoever coined that phrase centuries ago didn't live with a fussy baby like Nicki and I did. And how well do babies sleep anyway? My poor wife! Many nights Nicki didn't get more than three or four hours of shut-eye before Joshua's cries of hunger pierced the dead of night.

Joshua didn't start sleeping all the way through the night until he was a year old or so, and even when he did sleep longer, he never dozed past 5:30 a.m. Joshua was as regular as a rooster, always the first to let us know that he was officially awake at the crack of dawn. *I want my bottle!*

Sleep is a body therapy that's in short supply in the Rubin household, but I know we're not alone. A Sleep in America poll showed that children, across the board, generally snooze one to two hours less per night than they should for their age. According to the National Sleep Foundation (yes, there is one), infants between the ages of three to eleven months should sleep fourteen to fifteen hours in a twenty-four-hour time period. For toddlers, it's twelve to fourteen hours; preschoolers, eleven to thirteen hours; and elementary school children, ten to eleven hours.[9]

The Best Bedtime Routines

What are some of the ways to get your kids to go down—and sleep through the night?

These findings from the Sleep in America Poll conducted by the National Sleep Foundation may surprise you:

- Infants and toddlers who are put to bed asleep tend to sleep less at night than those who are put to bed awake (8.8 hours versus 9.9 hours).
- Children who sleep by themselves in their own room get more sleep than their counterparts who share a room or a bed.

- Children who fall asleep *with* a parent present in the room sleep less and are more likely to wake up during the night and experience nightmares.

- Children who read as part of their bedtime routine sleep more than children who don't read.

- Children with a TV in their bedroom sleep less than those who don't have a TV.

- As children get older, they tend to sleep *less* on weekends.[10]

How much are your children sleeping?

As for our son, I don't believe Joshua is sleeping twelve to fourteen hours in a day because his naptimes are hit or miss. I can assure you that it's not for a lack of effort on our part—or because we're letting him sip caffeinated soft drinks like Coke or Pepsi that would keep him hopped up. (A Sleep in America poll revealed that 26 percent of children Joshua's age or older drink at least one caffeinated beverage per day.) We've dealt with other distractions as well: my son doesn't have a TV in his room, is too young to play with a computer, and surely doesn't possess a BlackBerry, like his father.

Nicki and I try to put him down by eight o'clock, but that's hard to do since we always seem to have something going on at home. We like to entertain friends and business acquaintances at Chez Rubin for two reasons: one, so that we don't have another evening away from Joshua; and two, because we can enjoy Great Physician–type meals prepared by Nicki's well-washed hands.

Believe me, we know that children need adequate rest to keep them healthy and happy. While they are in dreamland, their bodies and brains are busy getting ready for a new day. Sleep releases growth hormones into the bloodstream and fights childhood obesity. Research has shown that shorter sleep disturbs normal metabolism, which can set the stage for insulin resistance, diabetes, cardiovascular disease, and obesity. Shahrad Taheri, M.D., of the

University of Bristol in England, said, "Sleep may not be the only answer to the obesity pandemic, but its effect should be considered seriously, as even small changes in the energy balance are beneficial."[11]

In the last few years, Nicki and I have become more and more cognizant of the importance of sleep in our lives. For one thing, Nicki realized how much she missed a good night's rest during Joshua's first few years. I felt unrefreshed as well when I woke up, especially when I volunteered to give Joshua his bottle in the middle of the night. We used to go to bed around 11 p.m. and wind down with a half hour of local news or catch a ministry program on Christian television, but those days are long gone. We're turning the lights out a lot closer to 10 p.m. than 11.

When that happens, we wake up feeling rested—and in better moods. There's an old saying: if Mamma gets enough sleep, Mamma is happy, and if Mamma is happy, *everybody* is happy.

Sleeping with a Child
by Dr. Fiona Blair

It's a question I'm hearing more and more in my practice: *Dr. Blair, what do you think of our child sleeping in our bed?*

Sharing a bed with an infant—or a toddler—is a highly personal and controversial topic. A practice as old as biblical times but unheard-of a generation ago, sharing a bed with a baby has become popular in some circles, even though it's still not a widely accepted practice. A survey of nearly 8,500 people found that 12.8 percent of infants shared an adult bed at night in 2000, but that's more than double the percentage in 1993, according to a government study published in the *Archives of Pediatrics and Adolescent Medicine.* Nearly 45 percent of those polled said they shared their beds with infants occasionally.[12]

Bed sharing leaves the little one vulnerable to being suffocated or crushed to death, but proponents say that sharing a bed encourages breast-feeding because when a baby starts crying, Mom is right there to feed her. Sleeping in the same bed is also said to calm babies, promote bonding, and give new mothers and fathers more sleep, although some parents say it's hard to find enough room to peacefully sleep when two adults and one child are vying for leg room and arm room. Sharing the bed with your child also puts a damper on marital intimacy.

If parents are insistent about being close to their infant during the night, I recommend they sleep in the same room but place the baby in his own crib or bassinet. Some infant beds attach to the mother's mattress. Keep in mind that adult beds are not designed with infant safety in mind. A baby can die if he's trapped or wedged in the bed when a deep-in-sleep mother or father rolls on top of him.

Sleeping with your children is also known as *attachment parenting*. At some point in their lives, children need to sleep in their own beds, preferably in their own bedrooms. Part of the growing-up process is gradual steps toward independence, and sleeping in their own beds is part of that transition.

Good Day, Sunshine

You may not have noticed it, but kids stay indoors more today than at any time in history—except perhaps when the bubonic plague swept through Europe's grimy cities in the fourteenth century. Mothers locked the doors and kept their brood under foot, a prudent thing to do since "Black Death" killed between a third and two-thirds of the European population.

Children stay indoors for very different reasons these days. During winter in much of the country, it's too cold or too wet to go outside; in summer, it's too hot. It's normal for parents to drive their youngsters from their temperature-controlled home to a temperature-controlled school in their temperature-controlled minivan. During the summer months, kids generally live inside air-conditioned comfort, whether at home or playing at a friend's house. Then there is the safety factor: working parents with school-age children prefer that they stay inside the home after school and during the summer vacation months.

The American Lung Association estimates that children spend 90 percent of their time indoors, which means two things for our youngsters: they're not outside in the sun, where they can receive vitamin D from the sunlight, and they're inside four walls, breathing stagnant air with two to five times the pollutants found outdoors. I'll address airborne toxins in my next chapter, but for now, I want to discuss the implications of children not getting enough sunlight.

Sunshine, as I mentioned in Key #2 on supplementing their diets with whole food nutritionals, is an excellent source of vitamin D. Their growing bodies need fat-soluble vitamins, particularly vitamins A and D. Vitamin A comes from animal sources such as eggs, organ meat, and cod liver oil, and from vegetable sources such as carrots, sweet potatoes, and most dark green leafy vegetables. Vitamin D, the "sunshine vitamin," is received from the synthesization of ultraviolet B rays of sunlight striking the skin, and high levels of vitamin D have been found to protect against several kinds of cancer, particularly those of the digestive system. Soaking in some rays attracts immune cells to the surface of the skin, which controls skin diseases. Higher levels of vitamin D in kids' bodies may reduce the risk of developing neurological and autoimmune disease like multiple sclerosis by as much as 62 percent, Harvard researchers report.[13]

Yet when children say, "Can we go out and play?" on a sunshiny day, Mom's likely response will be, "Did you put sunscreen on?"

That's understandable since millions of concerned parents know the following equation by heart: lack of sunscreen $\times$ sun exposure = skin cancer. Therefore, they slather their children's noses, faces, arms, shoulders, and backs with gobs of sunscreen, figuring the higher the sun protection factor (SPF), the better.

So can someone explain why, prior to the Industrial Age—when men and women scratched out a hardscrabble existence under an unrelenting sun half the year—skin cancer was basically unheard of? Why are we seeing a troubling escalation of skin cancer when we get *far less* sun today? (These days, about 62,000 cases of melanoma are diagnosed each year, and melanoma has been increasing in incidence by about 3 percent a year since 1980, according to the American Melanoma Foundation.[14])

I believe the rising prevalence of skin cancer is more related to our lack-luster diets—the lack of antioxidant-rich fruits and vegetables and healthy fat-soluble vitamins and essential fatty acids—than to our kids spending their summer afternoons making sand castles at the beach. The sun is actually our friend when it comes to cancer because our health benefits greatly from higher vitamin D levels. Dr. Edward Giovannuci, a Harvard University professor of medicine and nutrition, said his research showed that vitamin D from sunlight could prevent thirty deaths for every one caused by prolonged exposure to the sun and the development of a melanoma or skin cancer. All your children need is twenty minutes of sunlight a day to produce an abundant dose of vitamin D.

Having said that, it would be folly to allow your children to cavort at the neighborhood swimming pool without some type of sun protection. The prudent approach would be to limit your children's exposure to the sun between the hours of 10 a.m. and 2 p.m.—the time when the sun's rays are the most intense. You should reapply sunscreen lotion every hour, especially if they've been in the water. Use SPF 15 or higher, and don't be stingy.

At the same time, be aware that sunscreen doesn't provide all the protection you'd expect, and the reason why involves natural science. The sun emits two types of ultraviolet (UV) rays: UVA and UVB. We've been talking about ultraviolet B rays because they are the ones responsible for the manufacture of vitamin D in our bodies, but ultraviolet A rays are the ones that can do damage. UVA rays penetrate the skin deeper and are *far* more likely to cause skin cancer than UVB rays, which are 95 percent blocked when an SPF 8 or greater is applied to the skin anyway.

You, as the parent, should exercise common sense as well as your arms when you lather up your kids' faces and bodies with sunscreen protection, but please know this: sunshine is good for them.

Just not too much.

Do Your Kids Have Nature-Deficit Disorder?

A few years ago, our family visited some friends who own 180 acres of mostly undeveloped land surrounded by 750,000 acres of national forest in Georgia's northeast corner. What a great way to get back to nature. Even better, we picked all sorts of fruits growing wild and in their orchard, and their pristine water from deep wells refreshed us better than Gatorade ever could.

Someday we hope to return to northeast Georgia so Joshua can hunt for frogs in the gurgling streams or play hide-and-seek behind tall grasses with his new friends. Just as Nicki and I know that letting Joshua play in the dirt is important for his long-term health, we also understand that it's important for him to discover the natural world around him.

Richard Louv, author of *Last Child in the Woods: Saving Our Children from Nature-Deficit Disorder*, contends that children of the digital age have become increasingly alienated from the world of nature. The long-term implications portend disaster for their physical fitness as well as their long-term mental and spiritual health. Since today's young generation has lost contact with nature, having never been taught—or allowed—to engage in old-fashioned play, they don't know what it's like to squish their bare feet in a muddy stream, build a secret fort, or check out an anthill.

Louv asserts that paranoid parents have literally "scared children straight out of the woods and fields"[15] while shoo-shooing their youngsters toward "safe," regimented sports at the expense of imaginative play. The radius that children are allowed to roam outside their homes has shrunk to a ninth of what it was twenty years ago. But kids who "explore" their natural surroundings gain instinctual self-confidence and independence.

Fortunately, my parents were "back to nature" folks who encouraged me to check out the undeveloped areas near my home. I was too young at the time to realize that my parents were wiser than I once thought.

Water Sports

You want to know the definition of optimism?

It's letting your fully clothed toddler play next to the dancing water fountains at CityPlace in downtown West Palm Beach and expecting him to stay dry when the twice-hourly "water show" entertains locals and tourists.

Boys and girls have always been attracted to water and love getting wet. It must have been a hot day in the Roman Empire when the poet Ovid observed, "There is no small pleasure in sweet water."

The pleasure in water stems from its wonderful healing properties—physical and mental. Any parent who's calmed down a cranky child with a warm bath will attest to the therapeutic qualities of liquids. It's amazing how hot or very warm water improves blood circulation, transports more oxygen to the brain, and eliminates toxins.

Cold water, on the other hand, stimulates the body and boosts oxygen use in the cells. The use of hot and cold water in baths and showers is known as *hydrotherapy*, and it's as old as the Roman baths in Caesar's day. I'm a great believer in hydrotherapy and regularly take hot-and-cold showers, running hot water for a minute before switching to cold water for as long as I can stand.

I don't think Joshua is ready for hot-and-cold showers—or baths, for that matter. But I remember this from my days of swimming in the ocean: kids can stand cold water a lot better than adults. So if your children want to jump in a mountain lake fed by springtime runoff or swim in ocean water *way* too cold for you, let them jump in! Sure, their teeth will be clattering and their lips will turn blue by the time they get out, but swimming in cold water is very beneficial to their circulatory systems. And if you have a hot tub in the backyard, don't let a winter blast keep them out of the water. They can soak their muscles in hot water until they're parboiled and then jump in the snow and make snow angels. That'll create family memories—and be great for their health. Better yet, join them!

Easy for you to say, Jordan. You live in Florida. Okay, so I have a snowball's chance in Hades of making snow angels with Joshua at our Palm Beach Gardens home, but let me tell you about the time I went skiing at Vail in the

Colorado Rockies. After knocking myself out in the back bowls one afternoon, I did the hot-tub-and-snow-angel thing back at the condo. Talk about invigorating! That's something I hope to do with Joshua some day.

I also plan to introduce him to another form of hydrotherapy very soon: the sauna and steam room. When we constructed our new home, I splurged and had an awesome sauna installed in the master bath of our new home as well as a steam shower. Several times a week, I relax in the sauna and crank up the heat to 150 degrees. The steam shower is super as well: I can feel the tension and toxins pour out of my body through my skin.

iPod Generation

I think the Rubins are the last family in America who don't own an iPod or MP3 player. Well, we actually do own an iPod, but I have to admit that I don't know how to use it. I hope to pass my love of music on to Joshua someday, though, and when that happens, I'm sure he'll show Dad how to make that electronic gizmo work.

Music therapy is the use of music to promote relaxation and healing. I don't think Joshua will be interested in listening to lilting instrumentals or old-fashioned hymns—although he did watch "Baby Einstein" videos as an infant and seemed to enjoy the classical music—but I do know that soothing arrangements will improve his concentration and memory. I also see great benefit in his listening to contemporary Christian music when he gets older. He may not appreciate my favorite artists—Stephen Curtis Chapman, Casting Crowns, Mercy Me, and Jeremy Camp may be on the Christian "oldies" station by then—but I'm sure there will be new groups that he'll gravitate to.

He should recognize some of my favorite songs, however. When Joshua was a few months old and Nicki was having trouble producing enough breast milk to keep the little guy fed, he would cry to the high heavens. Nothing worked to calm him down until I had an idea one day: sing contemporary praise and worship songs into his ear. I was amazed at how calm he became. When he grew older but was still in his crib, we played worship music in his bedroom to help him fall asleep.

Although Joshua's too young to have his own iPod—and as a parent I would be concerned about the loudness in his ears—he's already been introduced to a superb body therapy in music.

THE GREAT PHYSICIAN'S Rx FOR CHILDREN'S HEALTH: CONDITION THEIR BODIES WITH EXERCISE AND BODY THERAPIES

- *Make sure they run like the wind and jump like jacks everyday. During the elementary school years, introduce them to organized sports like gymnastics, soccer, and baseball.*

- *Keep your kids moving by limiting access to TV and video games.*

- *Lead them in five to ten minutes of functional fitness before bedtime, if that works in your household.*

- *Pay attention to how much sleep your children are getting. They should probably get an hour more than you think. Remember that sleep is the most important nonnutrient thing you can do for their health.*

- *Expose your children to twenty minutes of sunlight a day—avoiding the hours between 10 a.m. and 2 p.m.—so that they receive enough vitamin D to build strong bones.*

- *If you live near the woods, undeveloped land, or common-area terrain, encourage your school-age kids to play outside with their friends.*

- *Let your children swim in cold or cool water, and tell them about alternating hot and cold water in the shower.*

- *You know the old saying: the family that takes a sauna together stays together. They are also a lot healthier. If your children are old enough, take a sauna with them at your local fitness club or home sauna, if you have one.*

- *Play worship music in your home and in your car. Kids soak up the melody and the words much more than you'd ever think.*

Take Action

To learn how to incorporate the principles of conditioning your children's bodies with exercise and body therapies, please turn to page 176 for the Great Physician's Rx for Children's Health Seven-Day Plan.

KEY #5

Reduce Toxins in Their Environments

I didn't know it at the time, but when I watched a nurse prick my left arm with an injection of measles, mumps, and rubella vaccine, the course of my life would change forever.

I remember my first vaccination clearly, because I was fifteen years old—and probably the only person at Palm Beach Gardens High School who hadn't been inoculated with MMR. I was immunization-free because my counter-cultural parents didn't believe in vaccinations. Dad was a naturopathic physician and chiropractor who loudly questioned conventional medicine's reliance on immunizing healthy children with vaccines prepared from live, weakened, or killed microorganisms to stimulate the body's production of antibodies as a defense against infection. He felt that vaccines weren't as safe or as effective at protecting the immune system as advertised.

When a measles epidemic broke out during my sophomore year of high school, however, the local school district issued my parents an ultimatum: either I submit to a measles, mumps, and rubella shot, or I leave school.

So I rolled up my left shirtsleeve.

Four years later, following my freshman year at Florida State University, my health took a nosedive. Like the Energizer Bunny running out of steam, my energy level felt as if someone had pulled the plug from the electrical socket. I was a counselor at a Christian camp that summer, and I can remember falling dead asleep anytime we traveled on a bus. But daytime drowsiness soon became the least of my problems. For someone who had never been sick his entire life, I was thrown into a battle for survival: waves of nausea, debilitating stomach cramps, painful mouth sores, and explosive diarrhea. As I've related in previous books, my health plummeted to the point where I was a walking skeleton—104 pounds of skin and bones. I barely survived two years of illnesses that nearly claimed my life.

Since then, I've followed scientific studies that hypothesize that MMR vaccinations increase the risk of developing digestive problems, like Crohn's disease, as well as autism. Although the research has yet to establish a clear medical link, I believe deep in my heart that my teenage vaccination flipped a health switch that sabotaged my immune and digestive systems. Until age nineteen, I had enjoyed perfect health and stellar fitness, so why did I have to endure two years of teeth-grinding abdominal problems that took me within an inch of losing my life?

Because there's considerable uncertainty surrounding the immunization firestorm, Nicki and I won't allow a pediatrician or nurse to approach Joshua with a syringe in hand. Our pediatrician, Roland Gutierrez, M.D., supports our decision. After speaking with him about our concerns with childhood immunizations, Dr. Gutierrez replied, "Jordan, I've heard who you are, and I am familiar with your books. I just want you to know that about 35 percent of my patients choose not to vaccinate. Although I recommend immunizations to my patients, I will still see Joshua if you choose not to vaccinate him."

I thanked "Dr. G"—as Joshua refers to him—but at the same time, I recognize there are two sides to the vaccination issue. Childhood immunizations against life-threatening diseases have been around since British physician Edward Jenner inoculated eight-year-old James Phipps in 1796 with cowpox to provide an immunity against smallpox, an acute, highly contagious disease that caused blisterlike lesions. In those days, the smallpox death rate was 50 percent or higher. During the nineteenth and twentieth centuries, an estimated 300 million deaths were attributed to smallpox until the World Health Organization certified its eradication in 1979.

Polio, which cripples the muscles needed for swallowing and breathing, swept across the United States several times during the twentieth century. My father was born in 1952, the same year a coast-to-coast polio outbreak prompted widespread hysteria. Children were warned not to drink from water fountains and to avoid amusement parks, municipal pools, and city beaches. Newsreels showed helpless kids locked inside iron lungs, which looked like a fate worse than death to frightened parents. The polio outbreak wasn't quelled until 1955 with the introduction of the Salk vaccine. Our country's first modern mass inoculation led to a 90 percent decline in the incidences of polio.

My father, like practically every child growing up in the fifties, was vaccinated against deadly diseases like polio, measles, diphtheria, and whooping cough. Called one of the greatest public health achievements in history, childhood vaccinations have prevented millions of premature deaths and saved countless more children from disfiguring illnesses. Well-intentioned laws were passed that parents couldn't enroll their children in public schools without an immunization certificate signed by a physician, unless they sought a religious exemption.

A half century later, though, I wonder if the pendulum has swung too far. Dr. Gutierrez told us that most kids get about *twenty* vaccines (against eleven diseases) by the time they turn two years old; that's a 400 percent increase just from the mid-1980s, when children were immunized five times against seven different diseases. The Centers for Disease Control and Prevention's current vaccination schedule calls for the following immunizations during the first six years of life:

- Hepatitis B vaccine
- Rotavirus vaccine (for infant diarrhea)
- Diphtheria and tetanus toxoids and acellular pertussis vaccine (DTaP)
- *Haemophilus influenzae* type b conjugate vaccine (Hib)
- Pneumococcal vaccine
- Inactivated poliovirus (catch-up immunization)
- Influenza vaccine
- Measles, mumps, and rubella vaccine (MMR)
- Varicella vaccine
- Hepatitis A vaccine (HepA)
- Meningococcal polysaccharide vaccine (MPSV4)[1]

Joshua has received none of these vaccines, and we plan to sign a "philo-sophical and religious exemption" waiver when we enroll him in elementary school. Nicki and I do not quarrel with the fact that childhood vaccinations have saved millions of lives, but we're concerned about the risks and side effects. Our worry is that one of these potent vaccines could spark the development of autism, asthma, diabetes, or developmental disabilities in Joshua. We are also dubious that the federal government is warning us about *all* the risks associated with vaccines, especially the new ones. Those in the know, including my colleague Dr. Blair, say the dirty little secret in the immunization world is that the way things are set up now, pharmaceutical firms use adults and children as the last "test group" following Food and Drug Administration approval for a new vaccine. We will not allow Joshua to become a guinea pig.

Why the Rush?

Gardasil, the first vaccine said to prevent cervical cancer, builds immu-nity to human papillomavirus (HPV), the most common sexually trans-mitted disease in the United States. A National Health and Nutrition Examination Study found that 3.4 percent of American women are infected with HPV, which accounts for eleven thousand cervical cancer cases diagnosed each year—and four thousand deaths.[2] After years of testing and development by Merck, the drug's manufacturer, the Food and Drug Administration approved Gardasil in 2006.

Young girls are the target audience for this new vaccine since Gardasil is most effective when administered prior to any HPV infection. Since teen sex happens, Gardasil proponents say the vaccine should be admin-istered before girls become sexually active—like the age of eleven or twelve. A three-shot regimen costs $360, which many insurance compa-nies cover but many don't.

Merck lobbied two dozen states to make Gardasil mandatory for all—repeat *all*—girls attending school, until dropping that effort in

2007. Texas Governor Rick Perry issued an executive order mandating the vaccine by the start of the school year in September 2008 for incoming sixth graders, but the state legislature rescinded it following vociferous protest from parental and family groups.

Two things trouble me about Gardasil: one, that Merck was donating money to targeted lawmakers in hopes that they would pass vaccine mandates for Gardasil in their states. At $360 a pop, there was a lot of money on the table if state legislatures ordered mandatory Gardasil vaccination for millions of young girls. Two, a mandate to vaccinate all sixth graders is grossly premature because we need more data on the vaccine's long-term safety and effectiveness before administering it to an entire population of middle-school girls.

There's another thing: I don't like how parental choice was pushed aside or the message that Gardasil will protect them from a sexually transmitted disease. That idea could encourage teenage promiscuity.

I am not a medical physician, which is why I appreciate having Dr. Blair look over my shoulder as well as contribute to the content of *The Great Physician's Rx for Children's Health*. When I asked her what she—a pediatrician who deals with this topic every day in her examination rooms—thought about vaccines, Dr. Blair replied that she has mixed emotions. "I do administer vaccines to many of my patients, but I have some who refuse them."

"Is that a problem for you?" I asked.

"I don't have a problem with parents opting out, and I support those patients fully," she commented. "But I have colleagues who will dismiss patients from their practice if they don't agree to immunize their children. I think that is short-sighted since we really don't know the full, long-range effects of the newer vaccines. I don't like to jump on the bandwagon the minute a new vaccine comes out. I usually wait one to two years before suggesting it to my patients."

I had other questions for Dr. Blair, and I think you'll find her answers interesting:

Jordan: What vaccines are normal in your practice?

Dr. Blair: By the age of two, young children should have received their primary doses of polio, diphtheria, tetanus, pertussis, *Haemophilus influenzae* type b (Hib), hepatitis B, and the newest one on the scene—Prevnar, which prevents infection by a bacteria called pneumococcus.

The Centers for Disease and Prevention recommend that we use a vaccine that prevents severe cases of rotavirus gastroenteritis, the most common cause of severe diarrhea in kids. Children often experience profound vomiting and severe dehydration from excessive diarrhea, but I haven't been inclined to use RotaTeq, a newly FDA-approved vaccine by Merck, at least not just yet.

Jordan: Why's that?

Dr. Blair: My hesitation stems from what happened in 1999 when Wyeth-Lederle released the world's first vaccine against childhood diarrhea, called RotaShield. Within the first year, a hundred babies developed a severe intestinal complication called an *intussusception*, which is an acute bowel obstruction. RotaShield was immediately pulled from the market. I remember deciding against offering RotaShield to my patients when it first came out. When Wyeth-Lederle recalled the vaccine, I knew I had made the correct decision.

Jordan: So that's why you like to wait a year or two?

Dr. Blair: When pharmaceutical companies perform trials on vaccines and various medications, they try to use as large a sample population as possible prior to FDA approval. They want to find out if bad side effects happen once in every 10,000 doses, 25,000 doses, or even 500,000 doses.

But the fact of the matter is that no one really knows if a horrible side effect is out there until the vaccine has been released to the general public. In a sense, FDA approval is the *last* phase of testing. When anti-inflammatory pain medications like Vioxx, Celebrex, and Bextra hit the market a few years ago, they were hailed as medical breakthroughs because they didn't have the gastric side effects that older drugs like Motrin and aspirin did. What we couldn't have guessed is that this trio of new drugs would cause cardiovascular disease, which is why they were pulled off the shelf.

My approach to new immunizations comes with a healthy dose of skepticism, but vaccinating children is definitely part of my practice. The vaccines I use are the tried-and-true ones that have been around for years. The polio vaccine is certainly one, as well as the one for chicken pox. That current chicken pox vaccine, called varicella, has been out for more than a decade and doesn't appear to have excessive side effects. I've used varicella on my own children, but recently the Advisory Committee on Immunization Practices and the American Academy of Pediatrics recommended that a second booster dose be administered to children who have not previously received the first one because the medical community is finding that immunity from the first vaccine wanes over time.

Another vaccine with a safe profile is polio, which has pretty much been eradicated in this country. It's still an interesting vaccine to talk about, though. Up until about eight years ago, we were giving polio in a highly effective oral form developed in the 1960s by Albert Sabin. The problem with the oral form is that around one out of 250 million doses would cause polio because the oral form was a live vaccine. In other words, we got to a point in this country where the only reported cases of polio were those caused by the vaccine.

Even though it was only one out of 250 million, if that one is your child, that's 100 percent to *you*. The powers that be, like the American Academy of Pediatrics and the Council on Immunization Practices, decided that was too much of a risk, so they changed the vaccine type to an injectable form, which is a killed virus. Your child cannot get polio from the killed virus, and the injectable form protects very well, although not as well as the Sabin vaccine, which is now only available in countries where polio is endemic.

Jordan: What do you mean by "doesn't protect as well"?

Dr. Blair: I don't know the specific numbers, but the injectable vaccine might protect your child 90 percent of the time, whereas the oral polio vaccine protected them 99.9 percent of the time. Since we don't see polio anymore in this country, we've decided to adopt the injectable form.

Jordan: But you aren't 100 percent for vaccines . . .

Dr. Blair: My issue with vaccinations in general is that we're trying to immunize children against the world. If their maturing immune systems are not fighting the viruses and the germs that they were intended to fight, then what will their maturing immune systems do? My suspicion is that their immune systems will start to fight themselves. I think that's one explanation for why certain autoimmune diseases—lupus, rheumatoid arthritis, multiple sclerosis, and even juvenile diabetes—are on the rise.

Jordan: Are parents saying yes to some vaccines and no to others in your practice?

Dr. Blair: I see parents wanting to do different things. Some ask for the full slate of vaccines; others don't want any at all. Others cherry-pick. I honor all requests, after we've had a little doctor-patient discussion.

For instance, some parents tell me they don't understand the need for their children to take the hepatitis B vaccine. They know hepatitis B is a virus acquired either by being born to an infected mother, through sexual activity, or through intravenous drug use. I've had mothers say to me, "My infant is not sexually active, and I know I didn't give him hepatitis at birth or through taking intravenous drugs, so why do I have to vaccinate him against hepatitis right now?" I'm fine with that thinking.

There are some parents who don't want the MMR vaccine because they've seen news reports calling it a possible source of autism. I, however, have seen no medical proof that measles, mumps, and rubella vaccine leads to autism. The concerns may be the result of the unfortunate timing of when we give the vaccine.

Jordan: Why is that?

Dr. Blair: MMR is usually given between the twelfth- and eighteen-month period of a child's life, and that's the same time the child starts to talk and socialize—and also the time when parents notice that something just doesn't seem right with their child. The baby stops talking or interacting. The social skills aren't developing the way they should, so tests are undertaken.

A formal diagnosis of autism is made usually between two or three years of age, which is devastating to the parents. Naturally, one of the things that might stand out in their minds is *Hmm, after he got that vaccine, he started to act this way.* So that's why the fingers are pointed at MMR.

Jordan: Role-play with me here. I'm going to pretend I'm a father of a child between the ages of twelve and eighteen months. I make an appointment to meet with you in your office, and our conversation begins this way:

Hi, Dr. Blair. I have my son, Patrick, with me, as you can tell. You mentioned at our last examination that he's due for several vaccinations. I've been talking to some friends at church, and they told me to think twice about the one for measles. I really don't know what to do.

Dr. Blair: What are your concerns? What kinds of things did your friends tell you at church?

Jordan: *Well, a good friend said she heard the MMR vaccine could cause autism, but that's all I know.*

Dr. Blair: With regards to the alleged link between MMR and autism, there have been studies that have particularly looked into that, but these studies have not borne any medical proof that the MMR vaccine causes autism. But we don't know everything, and I certainly don't want you to do something that you don't feel comfortable with. I will make this suggestion, if you're sitting on the fence:

If your child doesn't get a MMR shot between the ages of twelve and eighteen months, that doesn't mean we can never give it. I've had parents wait until the child is two, three, or even four years old for their measles, mumps, and rubella shot. By that time, we've established the child is developing normally, that the child is speaking and communicating normally, and that the child is socializing normally. All the connections in the brain are going well. But if you still decide that you don't want to give the shot at that time, that'll be okay with me.

Jordan: Have your four children gotten all the recommended vaccines?

Dr. Blair: Actually, they got all of them up to the chicken pox, but there are a few that I have chosen not to give them, including Gardasil, the new vaccine supposed to protect the girls from cervical cancer. I have a ten-year-old daughter, Courtney. She will not be getting Gardasil when she's eleven or twelve. Since the general public is the last stage of the clinical trial, and I don't want to be a part of that, Courtney and I are going to take a pass.

Jordan: Thanks, Dr. Blair.

I'm not recommending that you have your children vaccinated or not vaccinated. You can find horror stories on both sides, so it's important to talk to your pediatrician and do your research so that you can make an informed decision. In certain cases, there are real risks to consider. You have to ask yourself, why is autism, which used to afflict one in 10,000 children, now the scourge of one in 150 kids today? Why have childhood asthma rates exploded?[3]

If you're undecided, I urge you to listen to Mary Tocco, director of vaccine research and education for a group called Michigan Opposing Mandatory Vaccines. When she heard that the Michigan state legislature was threatening to remove the "philosophical exemption" and make vaccines mandatory for all children, she got involved in the fight to help stop the bill from passing. Since then, she has made the decision not to vaccinate her five children. Visit her website at www.marytocco.com. Another online resource to dig into is www.mercola.com. Just type "childhood vaccinations" into the Mercola search engine.

Homebodies

While Nicki and I recognize the benefits of modern vaccines, I still have reservations regarding certain immunizations and their possible toxicity to our bodies, especially when I remember all the pain and suffering I went through. But as you'll read in this chapter, there's a lot more to consider than vaccinations when it comes to reducing toxins in your children's environment, the fifth key to unlocking their health potential.

Thanks to modern chemistry, we live in a toxic world: for infants, toddlers, and young children, that world is usually contained within the four walls of their homes. Our offspring spend 90 percent of their time indoors, as I mentioned in my last chapter, which subjects them to around-the-clock exposure to numerous chemicals in large and minute concentrations.

From the air your children breathe, to the water they drink and bathe in, the toys they play with, the way you heat up food, and the household cleaners you use to keep floors, countertops, and toilets clean and sanitary, your children's bodies are receiving environmental contaminates that seemingly don't affect their health today but certainly could portend serious health problems years from now. You also may not be aware that you're unwittingly introducing toxins into their environment every time you wrap food in plastic, heat up leftovers in nonstick pans, turn on the microwave oven, dress them in jammies, rub polish on furniture, treat carpet with stain repellants, or spray the house with air fresheners.

Our homes are rife with chemicals that are clearly toxic or just plain harmful. *National Geographic* magazine, in a special report called "The Pollution Within," investigated what a typical house may have, room by room, in terms of a toxic footprint:

- **Bedrooms and bathrooms:** Foam mattresses and pillows, along with carpet and chair cushions, are home to polybrominated diphenyl ethers (PBDEs), which are flame retardants that cause developmental problems in lab animals. PBDEs are also found in children's pajamas as well as appliances, like telephones and hair dryers. The walls and ceiling could be coated with harmful lead paint. Kids' shoes could be smeared with fertilizer or herbicide residue from the backyard, or they could be exposed to a pesticide if they roughhouse with a pet dog wearing a flea collar.

  In the kids' bathrooms, phthalates are chemicals used to soften plastics and lengthen the shelf life of cosmetics, hair spray, mousses, and fragrances. You can also find phthalates in shower curtains, plastic bath toys, and vinyl flooring, as well as shampoo, deodorant, toothpaste, hair spray, and soap. Phthalates harm the developing testes of young boys and damage children's lungs, liver, and kidneys.

- **Living room:** Couches and carpets, as well as electronics gear (TVs, computers, and PlayStations) contain PBDEs. Your furniture fabric may also be treated with scratch- and stain-resistant coatings that contain perfluorinated alkylated substances (PFAs), which are regarded as highly toxic and extraordinarily persistent chemicals. Extension cords, vinyl wallpaper, and blinds contain phthalates.

- **Kitchen and dining room:** Some of the supermarket-bought meats you serve could contain polychlorinated biphenyls (PCBs), which are chemical compounds developed in the 1930s to make paint, ink, dye, hydraulic fluids, and common coolants. Found to inflict liver damage and cancer in lab animals, PCBs were banned in the late 1970s, but they're still being found in the fatty tissues of land animals and fish. Farm-raised salmon, for instance, are fed pellets of ground-up fish that absorbed PCBs from the environment. Mercury, a toxic metal, is also prevalent in canned tuna. Another toxic chemical known as dioxin tends to accumulate in the flesh of fish and shellfish.

  Nonstick pans used to fry up ground round or cook Hamburger Helper–type meals (God forbid!) contain PFAs. Phthalates and bisphenols are found in plastic containers and bottles as well as vinyl flooring. Coffeemakers, blenders, toasters, and microwaves contain their fair share of PBDEs.

- **Outdoors:** Step outside and take a deep breath of . . . ozone, particulate matter, carbon monoxide, nitrogen dioxide, sulfur dioxide, and lead, especially if you live in a city or suburban area.[4] There's not much you can do about clean air if you live in the Los Angeles smog basin or other metropolitan areas . . . except keep the kids indoors, which presents environmental issues as well since indoor air can be even more polluted than what's outdoors.

And then there's your water.

The water flowing from your taps likely comes from a municipal source responsible for making sure the water is safe for public consumption. Municipal water undergoes a series of filtration steps to remove fine microorganisms and dissolved inorganic and organic materials. Before treated water can be released from the treatment plant, however, it must be disinfected to destroy any pathogens that somehow made it through the filtration process. The most common disinfectant is chlorine or its chemical cousins—chloramines and chlorine dioxide.

Chlorine . . . yes, I'm talking about the white stuff the pool guy dumps into swimming pools so that nobody gets sick when the kiddies pee in the pool. (Chlorine, however, doesn't cause blond hair to turn green, fingernails to turn blue, or bathing suits to turn a blue-green hue. You can blame the buildup of copper in the pool water for emerald ponytails.)

Turning our focus back to municipal water supplies, chlorine has been the disinfectant of choice since the 1890s, when cities and towns across the fruited plain searched for something to combat water-borne diseases like cholera and typhoid. Chlorine was cheap and killed just about everything hazardous in the water. It didn't seem to harm humans.

The problem with chlorine is that it's a poison, low-grade to be sure, but still a highly toxic substance. You'll find out how toxic by letting your kids dump a large glass of pool water into an aquarium and watching the pretty goldfish rise to the surface—dead on arrival. Better yet, watch your dog lap up some pool water and see how sick he gets. Although humans seem to tolerate chlorinated water, it's hard on the skin, and if your kids ever spent a weekend at a resort pool, you may have noticed the way chlorine dried out their hair and caused a flaky scalp.

If your tap water is treated with chlorine—and it probably is—then drinking from the faucet, showering beneath a spray of hot water, or bathing your kids in the tub is problematic. When your toddler plays in the bathtub with his rubber duckies, the beading of the hot water opens up the pores of his skin, causing him to soak up the equivalent of several glasses of chlorinated water right into his bloodstream. The same physiological process happens to you when you stand beneath a steaming spray of shower water. For adults, taking a shower is the chlorine equivalent of drinking six to eight glasses of chlorinated water. Swimming laps for an hour at the local outdoor pool would be like drinking unfiltered tap water for a week.

That single hour is more than enough time for potent toxins to buffet your body, although potency is relative to the intensity of the exposure. Paracelsus, a Swiss alchemist from the 1500s, once said, "There are no toxic materials, there are only toxic doses," and technically, he is correct. Just fifty nanograms of botulinal neurotoxin will kill you rather quickly, but so will drinking too much water, no matter how pure. (A California woman, Jennifer Strange, perished after drinking more than a gallon of water as part of a radio show contest in 2007.) While drinking and swimming in chlorinated water doesn't rise to the level of a deadly toxin, it's still not good for you. Besides, the chemical aftertaste is horrible and doesn't compare to the healthiness of filtered water.

During the construction of our new home, we had the contractor install a whole-house, carbon-based water filtration system in our garage that removes the chlorine and other impurities in our municipal water *before* it enters our household pipes. We also have ultrafiltration and reverse osmosis filters at multiple sites in our home to further purify our drinking water.

Talk about one of the best investments you can make for your family's health. When Nicki's preparing dinner, she can confidently wash our organic produce in ultrafiltered water, and we enjoy the same peace of mind whenever we take showers, perform facial dips as part of advanced hygiene, brush our teeth, or plop Joshua into the bathtub. Drinking water from the tap tastes just fine.

The downside to whole-house water filtration systems is cost, which ranges somewhere between $500 and $5,000, depending on the size of your home. You also have to factor in the cost of replacement filters. Don't despair, however, since far less expensive options are available. Inexpensive carbon-based filters can be installed on your showerhead, but if you have the extra money, purchase a shower filter called a *kinetic degradation fluxion* (KDF) unit, which contains a special high-purity alloy that removes chlorine, heavy metals, and bacteria from the water.

I realize that most children, especially those under school age, take baths and not showers, so showerhead filters won't be much help. You can still give your kids a chlorine-free scrubbing and cleansing, however, by purchasing bath filter balls that float in the tub and reportedly remove 90 percent of the chlorine in the water. Another great way to reduce chlorine in a bath is to fill the tub with very hot water, warmer than you would want for your child, and let the water stand for twenty to thirty minutes. Since chlorine is a gas, most of the chlorine will dissipate within a half hour, leaving the bath virtually chlorine-free.

In the kitchen, it doesn't cost much to install carbon-based water filters at your kitchen sink as well as between the wall and the water and ice dispenser in your refrigerator. You can also find kinetic degradation fluxion (KDF) units for the kitchen. If you're renting and don't want to spend the money on a water filtration system, a modest investment of $20 to $40 will net you a countertop water pitcher that filters water for safe drinking. Lastly, you can take these steps to improve your water quality:

- Run your water for a full minute in the morning before taking a drink from the tap. "First draw" water in the morning is likely to contain more lead from sitting in the pipes overnight.

- Drink water only from the cold tap. Lead more easily leaches from the pipes or faucet into hot water.

- Boiling water allows the chlorine to escape, which could improve the taste of some heavily chlorinated waters. (Note, however, that taste is not an accurate indicator of the purity or safety of drinking water.)

- Buy bottled water. Many families choose to buy bottled water for drinking and cooking. Bottled water must be stored in a cool, dark place, such as in the pantry. Once it is opened, it must be recapped and refrigerated.

You may recall that "Thou shalt drink water" was the ninth commandment in Key #1, but let me amend that decree to "Thou shalt drink *lots* of water." When it comes to reducing toxins in your children's bodies, drinking water is one of the best resources you can call upon. God, in His infinite wisdom, designed our bodies to quickly get rid of water-soluble chemical toxins, but fat-soluble chemicals, such as chlorine, phthalates, and dioxins, are stored in our fatty tissues and can take months or years to be successfully eliminated from our systems. Flushing your bodies with copious amounts of water will rid your bodies of those toxins earlier.

So keep water bottles handy around the house, on car trips, and at soccer games, and remind your children why it's important to drink plenty of water. Let them see you reaching for a sip of water. Keep them sipping and sipping. That's all part of training them up in the way they should go.

Last One in Is a Rotten Egg

The biggest thing in backyard swimming pool construction isn't vanishing edge swimming pools—it's saltwater pools. Once an oddball exception a decade ago, pools with saltwater sanitization systems are part of a quiet revolution catching on in backyards from Rancho Cucamonga, California, to, well, my hometown of Palm Beach Gardens. Actually, try my backyard. When we were building our new home, there was no question that we were going to build a saltwater pool. I had converted the swimming pool and spa at our old home to a saltwater operation and said *adios* to the pool guy tossing pucks of chlorine into the pool to chemically shock the water.

Shock the water.

That's an interesting phrase as well as a linguistic reminder of how chemically potent chlorine is. Saltwater pools, using a filtration system developed in Australia back in the 1970s, have a salt-chlorine generator that automatically converts normal table salt (sodium chloride) to a natural form of chlorine that kills off algae and bacteria without introducing abrasive by-products. Instead of red eyes and flaky skin, as well as the pungent smell of chlorine in the air, saltwater pools offer crystal clear water and very low levels of natural chlorine salt. When your children thrash around in a saltwater pool, you can be satisfied that they're not sucking in chlorinated water.

A saltwater filtration system adds around $1,500 to the cost of pool construction, which is in the same ballpark as converting an existing filtration system over to salt-chlorine. From what I've been told, it'll only take a couple of years to earn back that investment since you'll no longer have to purchase those hockey pucks of chlorine.

A Body Burden

No matter how much we try to protect our children from environmental toxins, chemical compounds will find a way into their muscular tissues, circulatory systems, and bone marrow. If you had their blood and urine tested for various chemicals and toxins inside their bodies, you'd be in for a big surprise: lab technicians would likely uncover minute traces of toxins in their bloodstreams, including PCBs, dioxins, furans, trace metals, phthalates, VOCs, and chlorine. Scientists have a name for this chemical residue: they call it a person's *body burden.*

Preschool-age children have a much lower body burden than older children and adults, but we, as parents, should look for ways to cut down their exposure to environmental toxins *today* so that they will live healthier lives far into the future. One of the major reasons we've been so careful with Joshua's diet is because food manufacturers routinely add chemical compounds to just about every processed food, colorful candy, and diet drink invented. Monosodium glutamate (MSG), hydrolyzed vegetable protein, artificial flavorings, and artificial sweeteners like aspartame are examples of substances that overstimulate neurons to the point of cell damage and, eventually, cell death. We're confident that an organic diet of range-fed, pasture-fed meat and wild-caught fish as well as organic produce grown without the use of herbicides and fungicides is much better than commercially raised livestock and conventionally grown fruits and vegetables, which could have troublesome hormones, nitrates, and pesticides.

If only environmental toxins were as simple as choosing the right foods and healthy snacks to eat. I've already mentioned how we installed a whole-house water filtration system, but we're taking other proactive steps to minimize our exposure to environmental toxins in our home. For instance, we've placed several air purifiers in our home to circulate our "used" air through electrical charges to capture airborne particles, microbes, and molds. These days, many homes are climate-controlled by thermostats with maximum insulation and energy-efficient windows, which is great for keeping the house warm or cool, but the downside is that we're breathing trapped air that contains toxic particles. An Environmental Protection Agency (EPA) survey of six hundred homes in six cities found that the air was dirtier *inside* the homes than outside.

Air purifiers do an excellent job of cleaning up indoor air. So do house-plants, which absorb pollutants through their leaves and roots. We've strategically placed several houseplants, such as bamboo palms, throughout the house to help with our air quality as well as add to the classy décor. Houseplants such as spider plants, dracaena, English ivy, Chinese evergreen, and ficus are recommended for their ability to wash and rinse airborne toxins.

What about Your Household Cleaners?

Kids can create messes in a heartbeat, which is why Mom is always cleaning up something in addition to giving the house a thorough cleaning at least once a week: vacuuming the carpets, mopping tile flooring and bathroom floors, sanitizing the toilets and sinks, and dusting the furniture. (Nicki just reminded me that I can help out here anytime.)

Conventional household cleansers and disinfectants, unfortunately, are awash in VOCs—volatile organic compounds—that can cause eye, nose, and throat irritation as well as possible long-term health implications like cancer. These toxic cleaners may make your home spic-and-span, but they are also amalgamations of potentially harmful chemicals and solvents.

To keep our house clean, we use products such as vinegar, lemon juice, baking soda, and commercially available natural cleansers to mop floors, clean countertops, and deodorize bathrooms. (Dr. Blair cleans her home with the exact same products and says that she gets her white laundry whiter with a cup of vinegar and a cup of baking soda, better than any chemical bleach can.) Joshua's long past the crawling stage, but when he was sliding around our stone floors—we've never felt comfortable with wall-to-wall carpeting since carpet is a wonderful host for dust and synthetic solvents—we preferred that our floors be cleaned with natural products free of VOCs and toxic chemicals.

It's easy to find nontoxic household cleaners at health food stores, progressive markets, or online. Nicki and I are especially partial to Seventh Generation products, which are sold nationwide.

While air purifiers and houseplants are win-wins for the home, there's a common household appliance that's a big-time loser in our estimation—the microwave oven. You should have seen the cocked eyebrow from our general contractor when Nicki informed him that we were striking out a built-in microwave oven from the kitchen floor plan. Microwave ovens, which blast food with electrical and magnetic energy, really caught on with the American public in the 1970s, when lower prices made them more affordable. These days, 95 percent of American households have a microwave oven, and I'm sure millions of parents couldn't conceive of a world without the technological ability to heat up formula in fifteen seconds or meals-on-the-go (like SpaghettiOs and leftovers) in a jiffy.

My issues with microwave ovens stem from what electromagnetic radiation does to those in the kitchen and what that radiation does to food. Regarding the former, there's ongoing debate in scientific circles whether microwave ovens emit enough radiation to harm individuals or how much radiation one has to be exposed to before you have to worry about prickly topics like cancer. Until the scientific community and the federal government gets things settled out, Nicki and I will sit on the sidelines: we won't allow a microwave oven inside the house.

For those of you who wondered how we survived 2 a.m. feedings without a microwave oven, I can assure you that it took only three or four minutes to heat up Joshua's bottle of special formula using hot water boiled on the stove. That wasn't so long. The way I look at things, a century ago young parents would have viewed a cooktop with instant gas burners as something bordering on the miraculous.

I also don't like having my food "nuked" with radiolike frequencies either. When waves of energy bombard a plate of SpaghettiOs, for example, the agitation causes molecular friction to occur, which destroys the fragile structure of vitamins, minerals, and enzymes—not that SpaghettiOs contain many of the aforementioned nutrients to begin with.

A study published in the *Journal of the Science of Food and Agriculture* investigated various cooking methods of broccoli and concluded that microwaving was the biggest loser: microwaved broccoli had lost 97 percent, 74 percent, and 87 percent of three major antioxidant compounds: flavonoids, sinapics, and caffeoyl-quinic derivatives. By stark comparison, steamed broccoli had lost only 11 percent, 0 percent, and 8 percent, respectively, of the same antioxidants.[5]

I also don't think it's safe to microwave plastic bottles with baby formula or leftovers in plastic containers since this source of über-heating could release dioxins from the plastic into the formula or onto the food. (We also don't store leftovers in porous plastic containers or allow Joshua to sip from a flimsy plastic cup. Instead, we use reusable containers made from strong plastics and cups and glasses made of glass or ceramic.)

In our home, we rely on a toaster oven when we want to heat up something quick. I know that toaster ovens sound definitely low tech, but these old-school appliances do an awesome job of heating up homemade pizzas made from sprouted English muffins, baked potatoes, and leftovers. You can even cook a lamb chop in a toaster oven, although the clean-up is a headache.

You shouldn't braise lamb chops in a Teflon pan, though. A chemical compound used to make the pan's nonstick coating—called perfluorooctanoic acid, or PFOA—has shown up in trace amounts in blood samples taken from people across the country. Rats and mice exposed to PFOA in far greater amounts have developed brain tumors, prompting an Environmental Protection Agency advisory panel to label PFOA as a likely carcinogen in humans. DuPont, which has been making Teflon cookware and other products for forty years, says PFOA has been eliminated in the heating process that bonds the nonstick coating to the pan, but there's a lot of smoke around this fire.

Under scientific testing, PFOA keeps showing up on pots and pans as well as Gore-Tex jackets, carpet coatings, pizza boxes, and even microwave popcorn bags (which is another reason to toss out the microwave oven). Scientific studies, as well as lawsuits, are suggesting that nonstick pots and pans give off potentially harmful fumes at medium to high temperatures. This building wave of scientific research has prompted eight US companies, including industry leader DuPont, to virtually eliminate PFOA from all consumer products by 2015.

I know that nonstick pots and pans take away the drudgery of clean-up, which accounts for why 70 percent of the cookware sold in the United States has a nonstick coating, but you shouldn't wait until 2015 to change over to my favorite kind of cookware, which is made from enameled cast iron. Other acceptable cookware is stainless-steel, ceramic-coated, or stoneware. Dr. Blair is particular about her cookware, as well, and says that she's concerned about the safety of aluminum pots. Using cast iron pots, she added, is a way to add more iron to your diet.

You should also get rid of nonstick cooking sprays. Used in a variety of cookware—skillets, baking pans, casseroles, and muffin tins—cooking sprays keep food from sticking by forming a thin, oil-like film between the cooking surface and the food. The problem, as with most kitchen "convenience" items, lies in the ingredients. Pam, a popular nonstick cooking spray with an "All Natural" banner on the canister, uses canola oil and soy among its four ingredients, which earns a thumbs-down from me. The use of nitrous oxide as a "propellant" doesn't sit well with me either. I realize that ConAgra, the makers of Pam, have released a pair of organic cooking sprays, but I still feel it's far healthier to use coconut oil in skillets and frying pans or to grease casserole dishes and muffin pans with extra virgin coconut oil or organic butter. Better yet, your meals and baked goods will taste more delicious.

Potty Talk

If you figure an average of eight diaper changes a day, we probably went through 8,000 diapers before Joshua was thankfully potty trained. We thought about using environmental-friendly cloth diapers instead of disposables, which are manufactured with a chlorine bleaching process that contain harmful dioxins as well as certain dyes and fragrances, but Nicki said storing dirty diapers until the diaper service arrived a few days later would have done a number on her sanity. Still, Joshua had his share of rashes over the years, and we wonder how much of a role disposables played in that.

Maybe next time around we'll consider flushable diaper liners from gDiapers, which contain no elemental chlorine or perfumes. After changing your baby, all you do is drop the flushable part into the toilet. (The gDiapers have passed strict flushing guidelines set forth by the Water and Environmental Research Foundation, so it's okay to flush them down the drain. Check out www.gdiapers.com.) That would be a lot better for the environment since disposables are the third-largest single consumer item that gets thrown into the garbage, following newspapers and beverage containers. In fact, eighteen *billion* diapers are hauled off each year to landfills, where the untreated excrement may contribute to groundwater contamination.

Hide-and-Seek

Now I'd like to open up the bathroom cabinet in the kids' bathroom and talk about some of the things you'll find there and what steps you can take to protect your kids:

- **Shampoo.** Word association time: What do you think of when you hear about Johnson & Johnson Baby Shampoo? *No more tears.* That's because Johnson & Johnson was the first company to patent the use of a gentle cleansing agent that doesn't irritate a baby's eyes. Within six months of launching their No More Tears Baby Shampoo in 1953, J & J captured 75 percent of the baby shampoo market, and every other manufacturer has been fighting for second place since.

  Johnson & Johnson doesn't work for Jordan & Nicki, however, because the no-tear formula in baby shampoos contains anesthetizing ingredients as well artificial dyes and chemical preservatives known as *parabens.* We shampoo Joshua's tender scalp with something from Bronner's Soap, Avalon, or Aubrey Organics; these are mild baby shampoos with organic ingredients and essential oils. As for the "no more tears" part, I can remember Joshua crying in the bathtub for some reason or another, but never because his organic shampoo stung his eyes.

- **Toothpaste.** Have an extra box of toothpaste in the bathroom cabinet? Good. I'd like you to look at the small print. Search for the line that says, "If you accidentally swallow more than used for brushing, seek professional assistance or contact a Poison Control Center immediately."

  What's up with that? How are parents supposed to determine whether Junior ingested some toothpaste while swishing his teeth with water before spitting the contents into the sink? When I speak on this topic, I always get a good laugh when I inform parents that the red, white, and blue strips in their children's toothpaste aren't made from fresh strawberries, coconut, and blueberries, either. Unfortunately, most tubes of toothpaste you see stacked neatly at your local pharmacy contain artificial sweeteners, potassium nitrate, sodium monofluorophsphate, and trace amounts of fluoride ion.

  We've used natural peppermint oil-based tooth drops to clean Joshua's teeth. Our son will be making his first visit to the dentist soon, and our goal is that he'll go through life cavity-free. We think he has a great shot at that lofty goal since he doesn't eat candy or other sweets.

- **Sunblock.** In the last chapter, I talked about the importance of getting children out into the sunlight for vitamin D production and all the good that does for growing strong, healthy bones. Just twenty minutes or so of sunlight is enough for your children, but when you take your children to the beach or lakeshore, they'll want to play in the sand and seashore for hours. That's when your children need adequate protection from the sun, especially in summer, when the sun's rays are the most intense. The majority of sun damage occurs when children are young.

  To best look after Joshua, Nicki rubs Joshua's face and upper torso with a "green tea" sunscreen from Aubrey Organics that's free of petrochemical additives found in conventionally made sunblocks. She usually chooses the one with SPF 15 (since vitamin D can't be synthesized if the SPF is greater than 15) that uses titanium dioxide, a mineral that deflects the burning rays, as well as jojoba and organic shea butters as moisturizers. Remember, the skin is an extremely porous surface, and whatever you rub into your child's skin is immediately soaked in and spread throughout the bloodstream. That's why we go the organic route here as well.

- **Insect repellent.** We have lots of wetlands and stagnant pools in Florida, so the joke around here is that the state bird is the mosquito. It's not so funny, though, when a swarm of mosquitoes embarks on a blood-sucking contest on your kid. The itching is a major nuisance, as well as the risk of West Nile Virus and other infections.

  As is the story with sunblock, your children's skin readily absorbs insect repellant, which most likely contains DEET (chemical name, N,N-diethyl-meta-toluamide). Developed by the US Army for use in jungle warfare shortly after the end of World War II, DEET is a powerful pesticide. In fact, the makers of synthetic chemical insect repellents like Cutter's and Off! recommend thoroughly washing the skin with soap after use, lest DEET continue to be absorbed by the skin. The Environmental Protection Agency, however, says DEET doesn't present a health concern for the general population and has approved its use on children over two months old.

Uh, no thank you.

Fortunately, healthier alternatives are readily available. We like a product called Botanical Outdoor Gel, a certified organic aloe vera and green neem leaf extract that was recommended to us by Dr. Joe Mercola. It gives Nicki and me peace of mind and seems to keep those nasty mosquitoes at bay.

(Visit www.BiblicalHealthInstitute.com and click on the Resource Guide for recommendations regarding baby shampoo, toothpaste, sunscreen, and insect repellant.)

Lights On

Following our microwave discussion with our contractor, he didn't seem fazed when we informed him that we wanted full-spectrum lighting in our new home. Full-spectrum lights effectively emit the same kind of light that streams from the sun, as well as ultraviolet rays, which makes this type of lighting extremely healthy since UV light causes the body to produce vitamin D. Full-spectrum lights are more yellowish, which makes reading bedtime books to Joshua easier with less eyestrain. Our little guy seemed to sleep better at night after we installed a full-spectrum light in his bedroom.

One of the ideas catching on with the public these days is trading your old incandescent lightbulbs for compact fluorescent ones, which use about 70 percent less energy and last ten times longer. That's a great idea and one I certainly endorse, but installing full-spectrum fluorescent lightbulbs raises the bar even higher.

If you live in the Northeast, Midwest, or Pacific Northwest, your children may need full-spectrum lighting more than you know during the winter months when season-long cloud cover keeps the skies gloomy and gray. Reading next to a full-spectrum light desk lamp or light box can lift their moods and is said to be a welcome antidote for seasonal affective disorder—the wintertime blues—for adults.

Available at specialty light stores and Internet Web sites, full-spectrum lights may help you see things in a better light.

Artificial Sweeteners

NutraSweet, Splenda, Sweet'N Low, Equal, and Sunett remind me of the old saying: what's usually too good to be true *is* too good to be true. Sweetening a drink, cereal, ice cream, or candy with a potent chemical hundreds of times sweeter than sugar—with very few or no calories to boot—and not expecting health repercussions is like robbing a bank and expecting to get away scot-free. It's not going to happen.

That's why I want to end this long chapter with a plea to go through your house and toss out any foods laced with artificial sweeteners. Read the ingredients of any foods in your pantry or refrigerator. If you see any of the aforementioned brand names or words like aspartame, saccharin, sucralose, or acesulfame-K, treat them like poison.

These artificial sweeteners haven't been proven safe for children (or adults), and they never will. Board-certified neurosurgeon Dr. Russell Blaylock, author of *Excitotoxins: The Taste That Kills*, reviewed numerous studies on artificial sweeteners and concluded that not one is safe, especially for the growing brains of children. "If you feed your children off your plate or let them drink beverages and other foods sweetened with NutraSweet [or other artificial sweeteners], you may be exposing them to dangerously high concentrations of excitotoxins," he wrote, referring to studies showing the slow destruction of brain cells and neurons.[6]

Or the dreaded *C* word—*cancer*. Morando Soffritti, M.D., a cancer researcher in Bologna, Italy, headed a team that conducted a seven-year study of aspartame—sold under the brand names NutraSweet and Equal—and found in drinks like Diet Coke, Diet Pepsi, and Sugar Free Kool-Aid. His findings, released in 2006 to much media interest, found that the sweetener was associated with unusually high rates of lymphomas, leukemias, and other cancers in laboratory rats.

The Food and Drug Administration is conducting a thorough review of Dr. Soffritti's research, but this is another example of the dangers of consuming a popular food additive used by hundreds of millions worldwide. "If something is a carcinogen in animals," Dr. Soffritti told the *New York Times*, "then it should not be added to food, especially if there are so many people that are going to be consuming it."[7]

I can't see any good arising from consuming foods and drinks with aspartame or any other artificial—emphasis on the word *artificial*—sweetener. Instead, it's your parental duty to train up your child to enjoy the natural sweetness of a fresh banana or a summer-ripe watermelon. That won't happen if you're stocking the refrigerator with artificially sweetened fruit drinks or packaged treats.

R̶x THE GREAT PHYSICIAN'S Rx FOR CHILDREN'S HEALTH: REDUCE TOXINS IN THEIR ENVIRONMENTS

- *Investigate and study the pros and cons of childhood vaccinations. Talk to other parents as well as your pediatrician so that you can make an informed decision.*

- *Consider the purchase of a water filtration system for your home so that you and your family can drink and bathe in purified water. A less expensive measure would be installing carbon-based filters on showerheads and kitchen faucets.*

- *Improve indoor air quality by opening windows, setting out houseplants, and buying an air filtration system.*

- *Don't heat up food or drinks in your microwave, and teach your children not to either.*

- *Use natural cleaning products for your home, washing machine, and dishwasher.*

- *Use natural shampoo, toothpaste, sunblock, and insect repellent—or any type of lotion that touches your children's skin.*

- *Switch to full-spectrum lighting.*

- *Don't cook with nonstick cookware, which can give off potentially harmful toxins when heated. Cook with enamel cast iron cookware instead.*

- *Toss out any foods or drinks with artificial sweeteners, as well as those blue, yellow, or pink low-calorie and no-calorie packets.*

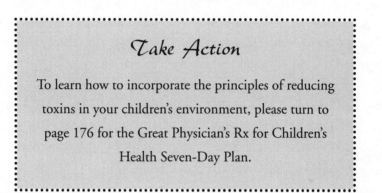

Take Action

To learn how to incorporate the principles of reducing toxins in your children's environment, please turn to page 176 for the Great Physician's Rx for Children's Health Seven-Day Plan.

Key #6

Help Them Avoid Deadly Emotions

It's amazing how life lessons have a way of staying with you. I say that because I've never forgotten something I learned when I was two years old.

I was a toddler, the first child of Herb and Phyllis Rubin. We were living in Marietta, Georgia, where Dad was a student at Life University's chiropractic college and working two jobs to keep food on the family table. We lived in a neighborhood close to school and several other chiropractic students. I can remember several of them bribing me with a toy if they could practice adjusting my neck. At two years of age, what did I know about being an "adjusting dummy"? I thought it was fun for them to collar me and give my slim neck a good tweak.

It's amazing, though, that these apprentice chiropractors got me to sit still long enough to crack a vertebra or two. I was a whirling dervish of energy who would have relished running Jim Thorpe's legs into the ground. One afternoon, Mom was cooking Spaghetti Marco Polo, which was whole wheat pasta with olives and spices. (My parents and I were still vegetarians then, so our diet was meatless.) Nearby was an old-fashioned water distiller. In case you haven't heard of these contraptions, water distillers produce disinfected water suitable for drinking, cooking, and other household uses. Apparently my parents didn't have great confidence in the municipal water piped into our home, so they used a water distiller to remove chlorine and mineral and microbiological contaminants by heating ordinary tap water to 212 degrees Fahrenheit, killing any bacteria or viruses that may have been present in the city water.

Our water distiller sat on a wooden cabinet that had a small door. I loved to swing like a monkey on that cabinet door, something my mother told me in no uncertain terms not to do. Being two years old, however, I had no comprehension of how dangerous it was to "play" next to a boiler filled with scalding-hot water, so I paid her no mind and swung on the door anyway.

I think you can picture what happened next: while Mom's back was turned as she stirred a pot of simmering tomato sauce, I jumped on that cabinet door for a swing. Suddenly, gallons of boiling water dumped on me, and I screamed bloody murder. I landed in a heap as scorching water flooded the linoleum floor. Dad, who heard my shrieks, sprinted into the kitchen to investigate. The boiling water burned the skin of his feet, even through his shoes, slowing him down momentarily.

I can't remember what happened next, but I'm told that my parents ripped off my clothes and hustled me outside. Dad grabbed some aloe vera leaves from the backyard and gave them to Mom to rub over me. Then he ran to the bathroom cabinet, where we kept various homeopathic medicines. He reached for a "rescue remedy" that he had saved for these types of situations, then hustled back outside and applied the homeopathic lotion to my parboiled skin. As you can imagine, I wailed to the heavens and cried my lungs out as only a two-year-old can.

Then my quivering parents wrapped me in a quilt and sped me to a local clinic for medical attention. I'm sure they expected the worst. By the time we arrived, however, I had totally calmed down. The tears had stopped. A doctor laid me down on an examination table, where he gingerly pulled away the quilt. Attached to the inside of the quilt were multiple layers of my skin. On my body, some areas of burned skin had bubbled and blistered, but what I remember is that I wasn't hurting. In fact, my parents said I was grinning from all the attention. I hadn't been administered any conventional pain relievers—just the aloe vera and homeopathic rescue remedy.

The doctor, however, wasn't smiling. After examining me, he informed my parents in grave tones that the entire right side of my body, from the face down, would be scarred for the rest of my life. I was destined to look like Two-Face, the villain and archenemy of Batman, whose face was gruesomely disfigured on his left side.

When I got home, my parents continued to rub aloe vera and the rescue remedy on my tender, pink skin. They also burst open pearls of vitamin E, which they soothingly applied to my burns. Their homeopathic approach completely healed me: thirty years later, my only scar is a dime-sized blemish on my right hip. You can't tell I ever suffered such severe burns, especially to my face.

I think my "getting burned" tale is the bedtime story that Joshua has asked me to retell the most, though he also loves to hear what happened to David and Goliath. It seems as if every time I trundle him off to bed these days, he says, "Tell me a story about when you were a baby, Daddy."

So I retell the story about Baby Jordi being in the kitchen when Grandma Phyllis was cooking spaghetti. Grandma warned Baby Jordi not to swing on the cabinet door, but he did anyway, and hot water came tumbling down and burned Baby Jordi's skin. At the end of every such retelling, I become very serious and say, "Baby Jordi disobeyed Grandma and Grandpa when he hung on the cabinet door. He got hurt."

I don't mind telling him that I disobeyed for two reasons:

1. That's exactly what happened. Mom warned me not to swing on the cabinet door, but I did it anyway.
2. I want Joshua to learn that there are consequences to one's actions. In this childhood instance, I was severely burned.

Early childhood is the time when parents establish their authority and set boundaries, and I'm trying to show Joshua what is acceptable behavior and what is not. I'm trying to teach him how important it is to listen to your parents. Mommy and Daddy really do know what's best.

Joshua has tried to stick his hand on our hot stove several times in the last month or so. Nicki and I have warned him not to do this. We've gotten at eye level and told him that he will suffer a bad "boo-boo" if his tiny fingers touch a hot surface, yet he continues to try. On each occasion, we've managed to stop him just in time, followed by a strong reprimand. Occasionally, we've rapped his fingers, but I can remember spanking him when we sensed his disobedience was based on defying us, not exploring his world. The reason I gave him a smack on his bottom was because Nicki and I do not want Joshua to burn his hand. We want him to learn to obey our direction because with hot stoves versus children's hands, the stove wins every time. When Joshua obeys, he's learning proper discipline.

When it comes to helping your child avoid deadly emotions, the fifth key that will unlock their health potential, the goal is to raise emotionally healthy children who aren't angry after being disciplined, hostile to your parental direction, or anxious about the future because they know they are unconditionally loved no matter what they do or how they perform in school.

Let's unpack the term *discipline* a bit. I'm realizing more and more with each passing day how important discipline is and why it's important to model this concept to my son. Like millions of parents, I've been greatly influenced by the teachings of Dr. James Dobson, who wrote the quintessential book on the subject, *The New Dare to Discipline.* Every now and then Nicki and I will sneak a peak at Dr. Dobson's book because we need to be reminded that when we have a nose-to-nose confrontation with Joshua, it's important for us to win decisively and confidently.

When I was Joshua's age, I thought I knew better than Mom about swinging on the cabinet door. She may have even spanked me after I disobeyed her and deliberately swayed on the door. I'm sure that she gave me a good whack because she wanted to protect me from getting burned in case I toppled the water distiller.

At the risk of sounding politically incorrect, I think that spanking is a necessary but unpleasant part of raising children. Dr. Dobson says when a parent administers a reasonable spanking in response to willful disobedience, the pain associated with this event teaches the child to avoid making the same mistake again.

Spanking is also certainly biblical. "He who spares his rod hates his son, but he who loves him disciplines him promptly," says Proverbs 13:24 (NKJV), and I take this Scripture to heart—not because I enjoy spanking my son, but because I love him. If I don't spank him when he deserves a swat, then the

Bible says I *hate* him. By disciplining him promptly, Joshua learns what the boundaries are, and inside those boundaries he has complete freedom.

Let me illustrate this by relating a story I heard about an experiment done at an elementary school. It seems that some voices in the school administration said the fence outlining the schoolyard should be taken down. *Kids shouldn't be fenced in,* they said. *They need to experience freedom, the idea that there's a big world out there waiting for them. Ringing their play yard with a fence is a harsh reminder that someone else is in control of their lives. You can see it every time they go over to the fence and look out. Why, some kids will even shake the fence to see how sturdy it is. They want to get out!*

That's how the thinking went in the administration offices, so the perimeter fence was taken down. But in an example of the law of unintended consequences, the schoolchildren did not flee the school grounds when they had the "freedom" to do so. Instead, they huddled in the center of the school yard, where they felt safe. Without a fence outlining their world of play, they didn't feel secure. Their boundaries were gone.

It's the same with discipline. Without boundaries defining what is and what isn't acceptable behavior, there's no freedom. When children grow up without learning what's best for them and what isn't, sooner or later they will experience a form of bondage. They will become trapped by their behavior, and when they make one poor decision after another, they build stress into their lives. In his book *The Pleasure Prescription,* college professor Paul Pearsall contends that young people today are *stressed*-out even before they get a chance to *start* out in life. He related the following story from one of his college students:

> "I'm always one of two ways," said an honor student in my psychology class. "I'm either tired and bored or stressed and maxed out. I only have two gears, high and low, and I think I must have burned out my clutch. What worries me most is that nothing seems really wonderful any more. I don't get really excited or really sad. I hardly ever have a good, long laugh or even a nice, cleansing cry. I'm going through the motions but I just don't seem to have emotions. I've been to Disneyland and Disney World. I've jet-skied, bungee-jumped, had

wild sex, been drunk out of my mind, and done drugs. Nothing turns me on or off. I'm only 19 years old—I feel like I'm in a pre-life crisis."[1]

That doesn't sound like freedom to me. Whether it's in diet, finances, or marriage—or a host of other areas that make up this thing called life—going your own way almost always results in terrible consequences. We see poor results when kids can demand—and eat—anything they want, and the parents give in, even though they know the sugar-coated junk is horrible for their health. The result, sooner or later, is childhood obesity. Type 2 diabetes. A lack of energy. Low self-esteem. The deadly emotions of resentment and bitterness.

It turns out that stocking your pantry with Twinkies and Ho Hos isn't freedom at all: it's giving your kids the tools to become overweight, unhealthy, and unhappy. Instead, you want to be serving your children foods that God created in a form that's healthy for their bodies, which trains their taste buds to prefer organic and whole foods over the junk that's so readily available. That's why your loving leadership—teaching them what they should eat, how they should behave, and what they need to learn about God—is so crucial in the younger years.

I've often heard that the first two years of life are the most important, and I've taken that saying to heart with Joshua. The emotional health of children is established early, and I know if we give Joshua a firm foundation in this area, he will be well served in the future. By learning self-discipline in what he eats, he'll say no when a friend offers him a Twinkie during school lunch. This self-discipline should transcend to other areas of his life, like how he handles his money and his future relationships with others.

I will not pretend that teaching Joshua discipline and order has been a piece of organic carrot cake. Joshua is a spirited child. He probes for our weaknesses and tests us on everything.

Joshua, do you want to take a bath?
No, I don't want to take a bath.
Joshua, stay in the bath.

No, I want to get out.
Joshua, put your clothes on.
I don't want to put my clothes on.
Joshua, it's time for bed.
I don't want to go to bed.

If you're the parent of a "terrific" two-year-old, I'm sure you're nodding your head in agreement. We happen to have a strong-willed child under our roof. But those are the cards we've been dealt, and we're going to do our best to stand up to his challenges to our authority. When Joshua obeys, he learns the meaning of self-discipline, and with self-discipline comes freedom from deadly emotions.

Is Unforgiveness Lingering in Your Heart?

One of the deadliest of all emotions is unforgiveness. Perhaps you've had a traumatic experience or suffered great emotional pain from someone in the past. Are there people who've hurt you so much that you can't find it in your heart to forgive them? It's a question worth pondering because I believe an unforgiving heart is an underlying factor in many health problems.

I witnessed for myself how a person's unwillingness to forgive can hasten his or her demise. For my Grandma Rose, unforgiveness turned to bitterness in the last few years of life. A European Jew who escaped to America with her parents in 1935, she never forgave herself for surviving the Holocaust when she lost siblings in Hitler's death camps. She never forgave God for the tough life she endured.

Grandma Rose married young, and her husband had a hard time finding a job, so young Rose had to work like a horse, performing menial jobs to keep the family going. Then her dying mother moved in with her. After that, a sister died, leaving behind two children, and those children moved in with Rose and her husband. Finally, I'm sure she resented the fact that her husband died of a heart attack at the young age of fifty-five, leaving her a poor widow for nearly thirty years, forced to live off a modest Social Security stipend.

When Grandma Rose had a second recurrence of cancer just before her eighty-third birthday, I rushed to her bedside, where I asked her to write down the names of people she needed to forgive. She wouldn't do it. She thought what medicine she took was more important than dealing with the people she needed to forgive. In the last six months of her life, I could see unforgiveness written all over the face of the grandmother I loved. If only she could have let go. If only she could have let God.

Please remember that no matter how bad you've been hurt in the past, it's still possible to forgive. "For if you forgive men their trespasses, your heavenly Father will also forgive you," Jesus said in Matthew 6. "But if you do not forgive men their trespasses, neither will your Father forgive your trespasses" (vv. 14–15 NKJV).

If you've had a long-standing grudge against a family member—and your children know it—let them see you make peace with that person. Whether you're angry, hurt, or bothered by those who've been mean to you, give them your forgiveness, and then let it go. Believe me, your forgiving heart will not go unnoticed by that family member or your children.

Children can be very cruel, which underscores the importance of teaching your children to forgive. I learned this the hard way when I was twelve years old. I was greatly persecuted by my Jewish friends when a man visited all of the local synagogues and warned the members to stay away from the "Jews for Jesus," whose practices he likened to witchcraft. Since I was the only "Jew for Jesus" that most of the Jewish community knew, I became a target. I was called a "fake Jew" and found swastikas drawn on my desk at school and graffiti blasting me in my own neighborhood. I lost most of my friends and was miserable. A friend of my parents encouraged me to forgive them, and I even kept a notecard with Matthew 6:14–15 under my pillow at night. Learning to forgive those who hurt me was a powerful lesson that would benefit me greatly later in life.

Laugh Attack

We've been talking about negative emotions and their effects on the body, but the flip side of the coin is that positive emotions, such as love, acceptance, and happiness expressed in laughter, are wonderful values to instill in your children. "A merry heart doeth good like a medicine," says Proverbs 17:22 in the classic King James Version translation, "but a broken spirit drieth the bones." A jolt of humor allows everyone in the family to forget an unpleasant memory. Laughter really is the best medicine for deadly emotions: this outward expression of mirth decreases blood pressure and heart rate while providing a boost to the immune system.

At three years of age, Joshua has no problem laughing, which makes him no different from millions of other preschoolers who lead carefree lives of fun and discovery. Children laugh around four hundred times a day, while grumpy adults find it in themselves to chuckle around fifteen times a day, according to the research team of Patrick Flanagan and Gael Crystal.[2]

As childhood obesity rates have soared through the roof, though, I think fewer and fewer children are laughing four hundred times a day because they are being laughed *at*. Childhood ridicule can inflict emotional scars that can last a lifetime. This was illustrated for me when I met Doris Bailey, a fifty-seven-year-old woman who attended one of my Weekend of Wellness conferences at Calvary Temple Church in Modesto, California. She's never forgotten the time when her brother and his friends laughed at her because of her weight.

The incident happened when Doris was just fifteen, a young woman trying to find her place in a big world but acutely aware of rejection and a lack of friends. She was diminutive in stature—just five feet, two inches tall—but carrying too much weight at 185 pounds. At school, Doris preferred to remain in the background, where she wouldn't be noticed—or rejected. "I was a loner, someone who stayed by myself," she said.

One evening she was home when her older brother, Sonny, a senior in high school, invited some of his buddies to hang out. The boys were cutting up and joking around when one of them caught Doris's eye.

"Hey, Doris, want an apple?" he asked. He reached for a shiny Red Delicious stacked in a bowl of fruit on the dining room table.

"Sure," Doris responded, not giving the question a second thought.

The boy tossed the apple underhand across the room, and Doris caught it. She had just sunk her teeth in the sweet apple when he suddenly belted out, "Hey, everybody, look at the pig!"

All the guys turned toward Doris, who was frozen in midbite, which only accentuated the image of a pig roasting on a spit with an apple in its mouth. Laughter erupted, which mortified the teenager. Doris ran for her room, where she fell on her bed and bawled her eyes out the rest of the evening. She fell asleep weeping in misery.

"What that boy said that night has stuck with me all my life," she said. "I never had a good feeling about myself before that night, and I certainly didn't think very highly of myself after that."

It didn't help matters that Doris grew up as an Air Force brat, part of a family that moved every couple of years to the next post. She always had a hard time making friends in places such as Madrid and Aranjuez, Spain; Hamilton, Bermuda; Palermo, New Jersey; Seattle, Washington; and Ceres, California, a small central California town where she went to high school.

Eleven days after her high school graduation, she married the first person who showed an interest in her—an Air Force aircraft electronic technician. When their first son was born fifteen months later at their posting in the Philippines, Doris was tipping the scales at 235 pounds.

Doris's newborn wasn't the only one gaining weight in those days. "I told friends that I was on the seafood diet: I would see food and eat it," Doris explained. "When we moved back to the States, I loved going to Perry Boy's, an all-you-can-eat restaurant, every Saturday night. I loved the variety of foods they served. I would skip the salad bar and fill up my plate with ham, bacon, fried chicken, mashed potatoes, and corn, making five or six trips through the buffet line." Her weight slowly but surely marched past 280 pounds after a second boy was born.

After twelve years of marriage, however, Doris divorced. She moved back to central California and settled in Modesto, where she met and married Larry Bailey in 1982 while working as a certified nursing assistant in nursing and private homes. When her weight crept north of 300 pounds, she gave up hope of ever slimming down. Sure, she had tried the popular diets—Overeater's Anonymous, Jenny Craig, and Weight Watchers—but they never worked. "I would lose five pounds, but then I would overeat a little bit or not follow the diet to a *T*, and get six pounds back," she said. "That was really frustrating."

Then on a Sunday morning, Doris was sitting with the congregation at Calvary Temple Church, minding her own business. I had been invited to minister at the morning services and shared a message about presenting our bodies as living sacrifices.

I challenged those in the audience that morning. "Can you say, 'This is the best I have, and I'm giving it to the Lord'?" I asked. "Are you an example of God's best? Can others see your vitality? Wouldn't it be awesome if God's people were so full of good health, so vibrant, that others would notice us from ten or twenty feet away?"

Doris didn't want to be noticed. She knew her health was far from vibrant. Decades of obesity had taken their toll: asthma, gout, osteoarthritis, acid reflux, high blood pressure, and sleep apnea. Her knees were shot: the only way she could walk was with the assistance of a cane or walker.

"I had never heard of you before you came to speak at my church," she told me. "When I heard you speak, I sat there in shock. The thing you said that made me open my eyes was when you urged us to eat only foods that God has created—not foods that man had created with terrible ingredients and additives or preservatives."

After I finished speaking that morning, she went home and cleaned out her cupboards and refrigerator, and then she went shopping for foods that God created. Doris began eating many more salads and either baked or broiled chicken. She stopped eating pork and sugary treats like jelly-filled doughnuts and apple turnovers. No more eating a half gallon of ice cream in one sitting. She filled her refrigerator with fresh vegetables, organic whole milk, and even some goat's milk and goat's cheese. She ate apples, bananas, or oranges as her lunch.

Doris saw pounds immediately come off—and stay off. What an emotional lift for someone who had tried every diet for nearly forty years without any sustained weight loss or health improvement. Now, two years after adopting the prescription from the Great Physician, Doris has lost around seventy pounds, going from 330 to 260 pounds. She's so encouraged to keep going that she's given herself a new goal: to get down to 175 pounds by February 2009!

Show Them Your Love

You want your children to feel secure? Then openly show your affection for your spouse. Hugging, kissing, and wrapping your arms around each other keeps a marriage alive and shows children the importance of contact in a healthy relationship. When Nicki and I cuddle on the couch while Joshua works on one of his wooden puzzles, we model a closeness that husbands and wives should enjoy.

When Nicki and I stand in the kitchen and happen to hug and kiss, Joshua wants to be right in the middle, not because he wants to disrupt anything but because he feels great security—a positive emotion—in our closeness. Sometimes, though, kids don't like it when Mommy and Daddy get all kissy-face. The older they are, the more they may say, "Yuck."

We expect that someday, sometime, Joshua will pucker his lips and say "yuck" as well. That's okay. Nicki and I will still kiss and hug anyway.

I sure hope that doesn't happen before he's out of kindergarten.

When it comes to helping your children avoid deadly emotions, always remain positive. If your children happen to be overweight, like Doris was as a teenager, your loving guidance and leadership in adopting the prescription from the Great Physician will help them lose weight and feel better about themselves.

℞ THE GREAT PHYSICIAN'S Rx FOR CHILDREN'S HEALTH: HELP THEM AVOID DEADLY EMOTIONS

- *Disciplining your children teaches them self-discipline, which will help them make wise choices in the foods they eat when they're older.*

- *Tell stories about when you were a child, which will bring you and your children closer together while imparting important life lessons.*

- *Teach your children to forgive those who hurt them, and set the example in your own life.*

- *You and your children can never laugh enough; it's your best medicine (Proverbs 17:22). Rent a funny, age-appropriate DVD for the entire family to share some weekend night.*

- *Hug and kiss your spouse when your children are present.*

Take Action

To learn how to incorporate into your family the principles for avoiding deadly emotions that I've shared in this book, please turn to page 176 for the Great Physician's Rx for Children's Health Seven-Day Plan.

KEY #7

Lead Them to Live Lives of Prayer and Purpose

This final key in the Great Physician's prescription for your children's health—although it's the shortest chapter—could be the most important, because one of the best things you can do for your children is to teach them that God has a purpose for their lives. And while you're at it, encourage them to be praying for that purpose.

From what I've seen during my limited time on this planet, many kids feel overwhelmed and wonder where they fit in. If they attend public school, they're taught that they're accidents of nature and evolved from primordial soup; the unstated message is that their existence on Earth will never amount to much. The ethos of the Sixties—"If it feels good, do it"—still lives on.

How sad! Each of us has been given life by the Creator for a purpose, not to do our own thing. I believe that purpose is waiting to be discovered by all of God's children. I'm trying to do my part by reminding Joshua that he's special in God's eyes as well as in the eyes of Mommy and Daddy. Because of his uniqueness, God has a very special life waiting for him. When I pray for Joshua before bedtime, I pray that he will come to know the Lord at a young age. I pray that God will use him to change the world. I pray that he will have the faith of Abraham, the courage of Joshua, the strength of Samson, the leadership abilities of Moses, and the compassion of Jesus.

Nicki and I pray regularly with Joshua because we want to model how he can talk to God. My three-year-old son hasn't quite gotten the hang of what praying is all about, but we can't help but smile when our little guy fervently bows his head at bedtime and says with all his heart, "Lord, bless Mommy and Daddy, AMEN!"

When I put Joshua down to bed, he often pleads with me to tell a story about "Baby Jordi," as I mentioned in the last chapter. If it's not too late, I'm glad to comply. When I told him the story about how I played the lead role in the popular musical *Oliver!*, I could see his imagination working overtime to picture how his father, as an eight-year-old, starred in a community theater production about an orphan boy who fell in with a gang of boy thieves.

Just before I leave his bedroom, I stroke Joshua's hair and say a prayer that's known in Hebrew circles as the "Aaronic Benediction," which is named after Aaron, the older brother of Moses and the first *kohein gadol*—or high priest. This benediction is found in Numbers 6:24–26. I love reciting the Aaronic Benediction in Hebrew. When I've finished, I repeat the Aaronic Benediction in English to Joshua:

> *May the Lord bless you and keep you.*
> *May the Lord make His face to shine upon you and be gracious unto you.*
> *May the Lord lift up His countenance upon you and bring you peace.*
> *In the name of Yeshua Ha Mashiach, Jesus our Messiah,*
> *Amen.*

I'm not sure what Joshua's three-year-old mind comprehends, but I really believe my preschooler understands a lot more than I give him credit for. Either way, it can never be too soon to declare that God will bless him and keep him, to make His face to shine upon him. The Aaronic Benediction is one way I'm trying to instill a purpose in my son so that he can grow up to be all that he wants to be.

Nicki and I also make sure that Joshua sees us praying—before meals, before bedtime, and sometimes on the phone when a family member or one who's hurting needs prayer. My great hope is that praying in these ways will help him develop a prayer life for himself.

Flying Home

On a recent trip home, I had a layover at the Salt Lake City airport with some time to kill. I meandered over to a gift shop and noticed several Delta

Airline toys in the window display. Since I travel a great deal, I sometimes like to bring home a little gift, so I purchased a small Delta Airline jet with a button that my son could press to make a "zoom-zoom" sound as the plane came in for a pretend landing. Like most boys his age, Joshua loves airplanes and knows that Daddy flies on big jets a great deal.

I presented Joshua with his new toy when he and Nicki picked me up at the Palm Beach International airport. As we were speeding north on Interstate 95 toward our home in Palm Beach Gardens, I watched him play with his new toy. "Hey, Joshua, what do you want to be when you grow up?" I casually asked.

"I want to be a real pilot for Delta Airlines," he insisted as he held the Delta plane in his hand and pretended to "fly" it, although I must admit, it sounded like he said "pirate" rather than "pilot." I also thought, *Boy, I must really fly too much.*

"That would be really great, son," I said. I'm sure that he sees those uniformed pilots with their classic navy blue coats, epaulets on their shoulders, and gold wings pressed to their breast pockets as superheroes. But I sensed this was a teachable moment to talk about what I do—my purpose in life.

"Do you know why Daddy has to leave you sometimes, Joshua?"

"Why, Daddy?" He stopped flying his new toy for a moment.

"Because Daddy's job is to help people who don't feel good get better. That is why Daddy sometimes has to leave you, even though he misses you so much."

I'm trying to teach Joshua that my purpose in life lies far beyond the material trappings of success. I feel with all of my heart that God created me to help transform the health of His people one life at a time. That is why I make the sacrifices I do: dealing with the hassles of traveling around the country as well as internationally to speak at conferences and appear on TV; preparing talks and writing books; and counseling others at conferences, on the phone, or by e-mail. God has called me to this work, and to those whom much is given, much is required.

My prayer for Joshua is that God will use him in a mighty way. Even though his young mind lacks the maturity to understand what I'm saying, I'm determined to plant the seed. "Joshua, one day you're going to do great things because God created you with a purpose," I said one time. "You're going to help people."

When I think about how close I was to death at the age of twenty, I realize that there was a very strong chance that Joshua could have never been born. But the Lord chose life for me, which means He has chosen life for my offspring. Because of His goodness, I have no greater purpose than raising my son and any future children He brings our way. Thinking of this reminds me of Deuteronomy 30, where God calls heaven and earth as witnesses to remind us that He is offering His children life and death, blessings and curses. "Therefore choose life, that both you and your descendants may live; that you may love the LORD your God, that you may obey His voice, and that you may cling to Him, for He is your life and the length of your days; and that you may dwell in the land which the LORD swore to your fathers, to Abraham, Isaac, and Jacob, to give them" (vv. 19–20 NKJV).

Whatever purpose God has waiting for your children, you have a great responsibility to train them in the way they should go. Your children should not be merely as good or as successful or slightly less successful than you are, but they should be better in every way because they can learn from all of the experiences that you've had. Your sons and daughters need to hear what you've done to overcome obstacles set in your way.

As Joshua grows up to become a strapping young man, I'll share the highs and lows of business, the good side and bad side of public relations, and the difficulty in sharing a health message with a nation that, for the most part, doesn't *want* to hear it. Learning from me will help him understand what I'm trying to do with God's purpose in my life.

As for Joshua, I can't wait to find out what his passions will be. Sure, we'll expose him to sports and music, but I can really see him becoming excited about the prescription for good health from the Great Physician. He may or may not follow me into the health and wellness field, but I'm not grooming him to succeed me. As New York Yankee catcher Yogi Berra once said, "It's tough to make predictions, especially about the future."

My attitude is that I'm excited to see what happens, although I know life may have some detours along the way. For instance, we know that Moses fled Egypt to the remote outpost of Midian after slaying an Egyptian, where he sojourned forty years as a shepherd of Hobab's flock. God used this time to prepare him for his purpose in life: freeing the Hebrews from their brutal existence as the Pharaoh's slaves and leading them to the Promised Land. Once the more than two million Israelites set forth from Egypt, however, they lost track of God's purpose for their lives. Their rebellion—and their unbelief that they could conquer their enemies occupying the Promised Land—cost them forty years in the wilderness, which is a very long time. I don't want my son to waste forty years, forty days, forty hours, or even forty minutes separated from God's purpose for his life.

You don't have any time to waste, either. Now is the appointed time; today is the day of salvation, Scripture tells us (2 Cor. 6:2). This sense of urgency should imbue you with the desire to share God's message of health and hope with our kids. Sure, you'll probably have to make changes in the way you eat, take nutritional supplements, practice advanced hygiene, resume exercising, and reduce toxins in your environment, but I can think of no greater investment in the health of your family.

I'm not doubting for one minute that you'll have to make sacrifices to adopt the Seven Keys. I'll never forget schlepping—a great Yiddish word—six half gallons of Joshua's homemade baby formula through airport security checkpoints before liquids were banned in the summer of 2006. You will have your travails as well.

I can assure you that the effort to change is well worth it, so my challenge to you is to go out and do it. Don't wait for your children to get flabby. Don't wait for your pediatrician to diagnose juvenile diabetes. Don't wait for another physician, evangelist, or health author to inspire you to make changes in the way you raise your children.

Instead, start that healing process today. Exodus 15:26 says, "If you diligently heed the voice of the LORD your God and do what is right in His sight, give ear to His commandments and keep all His statutes, I will put none of the diseases on you which I have brought on the Egyptians. For I am the LORD who heals you" (NKJV).

Now is your family's chance to experience healing. Go ahead: take a prescription from the Great Physician. May God bless you and your children as you travel down the path that leads to life!

℞ THE GREAT PHYSICIAN'S Rx FOR CHILDREN'S HEALTH: LEAD THEM TO LIVE LIVES OF PRAYER AND PURPOSE

- *Pray continually for your children's purpose in life, and let them see you praying on their behalf.*

- *Ask for God's protection for your family upon waking and before you retire.*

- *Be an agent of change in the lives of your children— today.*

Take Action

To learn how to incorporate the principles of living a life of prayer and purpose into your family, please turn the page for the Great Physician's Rx for Children's Health Seven-Day Plan.

THE GREAT PHYSICIAN'S RX FOR CHILDREN'S HEALTH SEVEN-DAY PLAN

Introducing the Great Physician's Rx for Children's Health Seven-Day Plan to your family depends very much on the age of your children. Because the needs of infants are so different from those of ten-year-olds, for instance, I have chosen not to produce a 49-Day plan as I have in previous books. The following Seven-Day Plan is not ideal for toddlers and infants, but if your children are older and you desire to make immediate changes in their health, I urge you to give this introductory strategy a try. Please know that you could have your hands full when you stop buying their favorite junk foods and start serving foods that God created.

Yes, this seven-day plan will involve huge changes for you and your family, but I predict that everyone will notice a big difference in the way they feel. If you wish to keep going after completing this one-week plan, I urge you to visit www.BiblicalHealthInstitute.com and click on the Great Physician's Rx 49-Day Health Plan, which is more comprehensive and can be adapted for your family's needs.

Finally, I am including the GPRx Resource Guide at the back of this book, which contains important contact information for manufacturers and distributors of products I recommend.

Need Recipes?

For a detailed list of more than 250 healthy and delicious recipes, please visit www.BiblicalHealthInstitutes.com.

Day 1

Upon Waking

Prayer: thank God because this is the day that the Lord has made. Rejoice and be glad in it. Thank Him for the breath in your lungs and the life in your body. Read Matthew 6:9–13 aloud to your children.

Purpose: ask the Lord to give you an opportunity to add significance to your children's lives today. Watch for those opportunities. Ask God to help you teach this principle to your children.

Advanced hygiene: here are basic directions that you can adopt for yourself as well as teach your children: For hands and nails, jab your fingers into semisoft soap four or five times, and lather hands with soap for fifteen seconds, rubbing soap over cuticles and rinsing under water as warm as you can stand. Take another swab of semisoft soap into your hands and wash your face. Next, fill a basin or sink with water as warm as you can stand, and add one to three tablespoons of table salt and one to three eyedroppers of iodine-based mineral solution. Dunk your face into the water and open your eyes, blinking repeatedly underwater. Keep your eyes open underwater for three seconds. After cleaning your eyes, put your face back in the water, and close your mouth while blowing bubbles out of your nose. Come up from the water, and then immerse your face in the water once again, gently taking water into your nostrils and expelling bubbles. Come up from the water, and blow your nose into facial tissue.

To cleanse the ears, use hydrogen peroxide and mineral-based ear drops, putting two or three drops into each ear and letting stand for sixty seconds. Tilt your head to expel the drops. For the teeth, apply two or three drops of essential oil-based tooth drops to the toothbrush. This can be used to brush your teeth or added to existing toothpaste. After brushing your teeth, brush your tongue for fifteen seconds. (For recommended advanced hygiene products, check out the GPRx Resource Guide on page 192 or visit www.BiblicalHealthInstitute.com and click on the GPRx Resource Guide.)

Reduce toxins: open your windows for one hour today. Use natural soap and natural skin and body care products (shower gel, body creams, etc.) for yourself and your children. Use natural facial care products. Use natural toothpaste. Use natural hair care products such as shampoo, conditioner, gel, mousse, and hairspray. (For recommended products, check out the GPRx Resource Guide, which is also available online at www.BiblicalHealthInstitute.com.)

Body therapy: make sure your children get twenty minutes of direct sunlight some-time during the day, but be careful between the hours of 10:00 a.m. and 2:00 p.m.

Emotional health: whenever you face a circumstance that causes you to worry, repeat the following: "Lord, I trust You. I cast my cares upon You, and I believe that You're going to take care of [insert your current situation] and make my health and my body strong." Teach your children this prayer.

Breakfast

Make a smoothie in a blender with the following ingredients:

1 cup plain yogurt or kefir (sheep's or goat's milk is best)

1 tablespoon organic flaxseed oil

1 tablespoon organic raw honey

1 cup organic fruit (berries, banana, peaches, pineapple, etc.)

2 tablespoons goat's milk protein powder (for recommended products, check out the GPRx Resource Guide on page 192 or visit www.BiblicalHealthInstitute.com and click on the GPRx Resource Guide)

dash of vanilla extract (optional)

½ teaspoon of children's probiotic powder (for recommended products, check out the GPRx Resource Guide on page 192, or visit www.BiblicalHealthInstitute.com and click on the GPRx Resource Guide)

Remember: this recipe serves one to three children.

Lunch

During lunch, have everyone drink four to eight ounces of water.

turkey and goat cheese on sprouted tortilla

carrot and celery sticks

one apple with skin

Dinner

During dinner, have everyone drink four to eight ounces of water.

baked, poached, or grilled wild-caught salmon

steamed broccoli

green salad with mixed greens, avocado, carrots, cucumbers, celery, tomato, red cabbage, red onions, red peppers, and sprouts (feel free to eliminate vegetables like cabbage, peppers, and onions if your children won't eat them at this time)

salad dressing: extra virgin olive oil, apple cider vinegar or lemon juice, Celtic Sea Salt, herbs, and spices; or, mix one tablespoon of extra virgin olive oil with one table-spoon of a healthy store-bought dressing

Supplements: serve your children one or two teaspoons of a high omega-3 cod liver oil complex (for recommended products, check out the GPRx Resource Guide on page 192 or visit www.BiblicalHealthInstitute.com and click on the GPRx Resource Guide).

Snacks

Have your children drink four to eight ounces of water, or hot or iced fresh-brewed tea with honey.

apple slices with raw almond butter

half of a whole food nutrition bar with beta-glucans from soluble oat fiber (for recommended products, check out the GPRx Resource Guide, which is also available online at www.BiblicalHealthInstitute.com)

Before Bed

Exercise: go for a walk outdoors with your children or participate in a favorite sport or recreational activity.

Body therapy: give your children a warm bath for fifteen minutes with eight drops of biblical essential oils added.

Advanced hygiene: repeat the advanced hygiene instructions from the morning of Day 1.

Prayer: thank God for this day, asking Him to give your children a restoring night's rest and a fresh start tomorrow. Thank Him for His steadfast love that never ceases and His mercies, new every morning. Read Romans 8:35, 37–39 aloud to your children.

Sleep: get everyone to bed fifteen minutes earlier than usual.

DAY 2

Upon Waking

Prayer: thank God because this is the day that the Lord has made. Rejoice and be glad in it. Thank Him for the breath in your lungs and the life in your body. Read Psalm 91 aloud to your children.

Purpose: ask the Lord to give your children an opportunity to add significance to someone's life today.

Advanced hygiene: follow the advanced hygiene recommendations from the morning of Day 1.

Reduce toxins: follow the recommendations to reduce toxins from the morning of Day 1.

Emotional health: follow the emotional health recommendations from the morning of Day 1.

Breakfast

one or two eggs any style, cooked in one tablespoon of extra virgin coconut oil (for recommended products, check out the GPRx Resource Guide, which is also available online at www.BiblicalHealthInstitute.com)

stir-fried onions, mushrooms, and peppers

one slice of sprouted or yeast-free whole grain bread with almond butter and honey

Supplements: serve each child a half teaspoon of a children's probiotic powder mixed in water or juice.

Lunch

During lunch, have everyone drink four to eight ounces of water.

low-mercury, high omega-3 tuna on sprouted or yeast-free whole grain bread with lettuce, tomato, and sprouts

organic grapes

Dinner

During dinner, have everyone drink four to eight ounces of water.

roasted organic chicken

cooked vegetables (carrots, onions, peas, etc.)

green salad with mixed greens, avocado, carrots, tomato, red cabbage, red onions, red peppers, and sprouts (feel free to eliminate vegetables like cabbage, peppers, and onions if your children won't eat them at this time)

salad dressing: extra virgin olive oil, apple cider vinegar or lemon juice, Celtic Sea Salt, herbs, and spices; or, mix one tablespoon of extra virgin olive oil with one table-spoon of a healthy store-bought dressing

Supplements: serve your children one or two teaspoons of a high omega-3 cod liver oil complex.

Snacks

Have everyone drink four to twelve ounces of water, or hot or iced fresh-brewed tea with honey.

raw almonds and apple wedges

half of a whole food nutrition bar with beta-glucans from soluble oat fiber

Before Bed

Exercise: go for a walk outdoors, jump on a mini-trampoline with your children, or participate in a favorite sport or recreational activity.

Advanced hygiene: repeat the advanced hygiene instructions from the morning of Day 1.

Prayer: thank God for this day, asking Him to give your children a restoring night's rest and a fresh start tomorrow. Thank Him for His steadfast love that never ceases and His mercies, new every morning. Read 1 Corinthians 13:4–8 aloud to your children.

Body therapy: let the kids spend ten minutes listening to soothing music before they fall asleep.

Sleep: get everyone to bed fifteen minutes earlier than usual.

Day 3

Upon Waking

Prayer: thank God because this is the day that the Lord has made. Rejoice and be glad in it. Thank Him for the breath in your lungs and the life in your body. Read Ephesians 6:13–18 aloud to your children.

Purpose: ask the Lord to give your children an opportunity to add significance to someone's life today. Watch for that opportunity.

Advanced hygiene: follow the advanced hygiene recommendations from the morning of Day 1.

Reduce toxins: follow the recommendations to reduce toxins from the morning of Day 1.

Body therapy: make sure your children get twenty minutes of direct sunlight sometime during the day, but be careful between the hours of 10:00 a.m. and 2:00 p.m.

Emotional health: follow the emotional health recommendations from Day 1.

Breakfast

four to six ounces of organic whole milk yogurt or cottage cheese with fruit (pineapple, peaches, or berries), honey, and a dash of vanilla extract

a piece of sprouted whole wheat toast with organic butter

Supplements: serve each child a half teaspoon of a children's probiotic powder in water or juice.

Lunch

During lunch, have everyone drink four to eight ounces of water.

turkey on sprouted or yeast-free whole grain bread with lettuce, tomato, and sprouts

one piece of fruit in season

Dinner

During dinner, have everyone drink four to eight ounces of water.

red meat steak (beef, buffalo, or venison)

steamed broccoli

baked sweet potato with butter

green salad with mixed greens, avocado, carrots, cucumbers, celery, tomatoes, red cabbage, red peppers, red onions, and sprouts (feel free to eliminate vegetables like cabbage, peppers, and onions if your children won't eat them at this time)

salad dressing: extra virgin olive oil, apple cider vinegar or lemon juice, Celtic Sea

Salt, herbs, and spices; or, mix one tablespoon of extra virgin olive oil with one tablespoon of a healthy store-bought dressing

Supplements: serve your kids one or two teaspoons of a high omega-3 cod liver oil complex.

Snacks

Have everyone drink four to eight ounces of water.

raisins and almonds

one half of a berry antioxidant whole food nutrition bar with beta-glucans from soluble oat fiber

Before Bed

Exercise: go for a walk outdoors with your children or participate in a favorite sport or recreational activity.

Body therapy: give your children a warm bath for fifteen minutes with eight drops of biblical essential oils added.

Advanced hygiene: follow the advanced hygiene instructions from the morning of Day 1.

Prayer: thank God for this day, asking Him to give your children a restoring night's rest and a fresh start tomorrow. Thank Him for His steadfast love that never ceases and His mercies, new every morning. Read Philippians 4:4–8, 11–13, 19 aloud to your children.

Sleep: get everyone to bed fifteen minutes earlier than usual.

Day 4

Upon Waking

Prayer: thank God because this is the day that the Lord has made. Rejoice and be glad in it. Thank Him for the breath in your lungs and the life in your body. Read Matthew 6:9–13 aloud.

Purpose: ask the Lord to give your children an opportunity to add significance to someone's life today. Watch for that opportunity. Ask God to use them this day for His intended purpose.

Advanced hygiene: follow the advanced hygiene recommendations from Day 1.

Reduce toxins: follow the recommendations for reducing toxins from Day 1.

Emotional health: follow the emotional health recommendations from the morning of Day 1.

Breakfast

one or two soft-boiled or poached eggs

four ounces of sprouted whole grain cereal with two ounces of whole milk yogurt (for recommended products, check out the GPRx Resource Guide, which is also available online at www.BiblicalHealthInstitute.com)

Supplements: serve each child a half teaspoon of a children's probiotic with water or juice.

Lunch

During lunch, have everyone drink four to eight ounces of water.

Chicken Soup (you can find this recipe as well as 250 other healthy and delicious recipes by visiting www.BiblicalHealthInstitutes.com)

one bunch of grapes with seeds

Dinner

During dinner, have everyone drink four to eight ounces of water.

grilled chicken breast

steamed veggies

small portion of non-gluten whole grain (quinoa, amaranth, millet, or buckwheat) cooked with one tablespoon of extra virgin coconut oil

green salad with mixed greens, avocado, carrots, cucumbers, celery, tomatoes, red cabbage, red peppers, red onions, and sprouts (feel free to eliminate vegetables like cabbage, peppers, and onions if your children won't eat them at this time)

salad dressing: extra virgin olive oil, apple cider vinegar or lemon juice, Celtic Sea Salt, herbs, and spices; or, mix one tablespoon of extra virgin olive oil with one tablespoon of a healthy store-bought dressing

Supplements: serve the kids one or two teaspoons of a high omega-3 cod liver oil complex.

Snacks

Have everyone drink four to eight ounces of water, or hot or iced fresh-brewed tea with honey.

apple and carrots with raw almond butter

one half of a berry antioxidant whole food nutrition bar with beta glucans from soluble oat fiber

Before Bed

Have everyone drink four to twelve ounces of water.

Exercise: go for a walk outdoors with your children or participate in a favorite sport or recreational activity.

Advanced hygiene: follow the advanced hygiene recommendations from the morning of Day 1.

Prayer: thank God for this day, asking Him to give your children a restoring night's rest and a fresh start tomorrow. Thank Him for His steadfast love that never ceases and His mercies that are new every morning. Read Romans 8:35, 37–39 aloud to your children.

Body therapy: let your children spend ten minutes listening to soothing music before they fall asleep.

Sleep: get everyone to bed fifteen minutes earlier than usual.

Day 5

Upon Waking

Prayer: thank God because this is the day that the Lord has made. Rejoice and be glad in it. Thank Him for the breath in your lungs and the life in your body. Read Isaiah 58:6–9 aloud to your children.

Purpose: ask the Lord to give your children an opportunity to add significance to someone's life today. Watch for that opportunity.

Advanced hygiene: follow the advanced hygiene recommendations from Day 1.

Reduce toxins: follow the recommendations for reducing toxins from Day 1.

Body therapy: make sure your children get twenty minutes of direct sunlight sometime during the day, but be careful between the hours of 10:00 a.m. and 2:00 p.m.

Emotional health: follow the emotional health recommendations from the morning of Day 1.

Breakfast

For a healthy smoothie, mix the following in a blender:

eight ounces plain whole milk, yogurt, or kefir

1 tablespoon honey

½ cup fresh or frozen fruit (bananas, peaches, berries, pineapple, etc.)

1 teaspoon high-lignan flaxseed oil

1 serving of goat's milk protein powder

½ teaspoon of children's probiotic powder

Lunch

During lunch, have everyone drink four to eight ounces of water.

turkey on sprouted or yeast-free whole grain bread with lettuce, tomato, and sprouts

one piece of fruit

Dinner

During dinner, have everyone drink four to eight ounces of water.

Spinach and Goat Cheese Meat Lasagna (visit www.BiblicalHealthInsitute.com for the recipe)

green salad with mixed greens, avocado, carrots, cucumbers, celery, tomatoes, red cabbage, red peppers, red onions, and sprouts (feel free to eliminate vegetables like cabbage, peppers, and onions if your children won't eat them at this time)

salad dressing: extra virgin olive oil, apple cider vinegar or lemon juice, Celtic Sea Salt, herbs, and spices; or, mix one tablespoon of extra virgin olive oil with one tablespoon of a healthy store-bought dressing

Supplements: serve your children one or two teaspoons of a high omega-3 cod liver oil complex.

Snacks

one half of an apple cinnamon fiber whole food bar (with beta-glucans from soluble oat fiber)

Zesty Popcorn with butter and spices (visit www.BiblicalHealthInstitute.com for the recipe)

Before Bed

Exercise: go for a walk outdoors with your children or participate in a favorite sport or recreational activity.

Advanced hygiene: follow the advanced hygiene recommendations from the morning of Day 1.

Body therapy: give the kids a warm bath for fifteen minutes with eight drops of biblical essential oils added.

Prayer: thank God for this day, asking Him to give your children a restoring night's rest and a fresh start tomorrow. Thank Him for His steadfast love that never ceases and His mercies that are new every morning. Read Isaiah 58:6–9 aloud to your children.

Sleep: get everyone to bed fifteen minutes earlier than usual.

Day 6

Upon Waking

Prayer: thank God because this is the day that the Lord has made. Rejoice and be glad in it. Thank Him for the breath in your lungs and the life in your body. Read Psalm 23 aloud to your children.

Purpose: ask the Lord to give your children an opportunity to add significance to someone's life today. Watch for that opportunity.

Advanced hygiene: follow the advanced hygiene recommendations from Day 1.

Reduce toxins: follow the recommendations for reducing toxins from Day 1.

Body therapy: make sure your children get twenty minutes of direct sunlight sometime during the day, but be careful between the hours of 10:00 a.m. and 2:00 p.m.

Emotional health: follow the emotional health recommendations from the morning of Day 1.

Breakfast

two or three eggs cooked any style in one tablespoon of extra virgin coconut oil

one grapefruit or orange

Supplements: serve each child a half teaspoon of a children's probiotic powder in water or juice.

Lunch

During lunch, have everyone drink four to eight ounces of water.

low-mercury, high omega-3 tuna on sprouted or yeast-free whole grain bread with lettuce, tomato, and sprouts

one organic apple with the skin

Dinner

During dinner, have everyone drink four to eight ounces of water.

fish of choice

brown rice

green salad with mixed greens, carrots, cucumbers, celery, tomatoes, red cabbage, red peppers, red onions, and sprouts (feel free to eliminate vegetables like cabbage, peppers, and onions if your children won't eat them at this time)

salad dressing: extra virgin olive oil, apple cider vinegar or lemon juice, Celtic Sea Salt, herbs, and spices; or, mix one tablespoon of extra virgin olive oil with one tablespoon of a healthy store-bought dressing

Supplements: serve the children one or two teaspoons of a high omega-3 cod liver oil complex.

Snacks

Have everyone drink four to eight ounces of water.

cottage cheese, honey, and berries

one half of a berry antioxidant whole food nutrition bar with beta-glucans from soluble oat fiber

Before Bed

Exercise: go for a walk outdoors with your children or participate in a favorite sport or recreational activity.

Advanced hygiene: follow the advanced hygiene recommendations from the morning of Day 1.

Prayer: thank God for this day, asking Him to give your children a restoring night's rest and a fresh start tomorrow. Thank Him for His steadfast love that never ceases and His mercies that are new every morning. Read Psalm 23 aloud.

Body therapy: let the kids spend ten minutes listening to soothing music before they fall asleep.

Sleep: get everyone to bed fifteen minutes earlier than usual.

DAY 7

Upon Waking

Prayer: thank God because this is the day that the Lord has made. Rejoice and be glad in it. Thank Him for the breath in your lungs and the life in your body. Read Psalm 91 aloud to your children.

Purpose: ask the Lord to give your children an opportunity to add significance to someone's life today. Watch for that opportunity. Ask God to help you teach this principle to your children.

Advanced hygiene: follow the advanced hygiene recommendations from Day 1.

Reduce toxins: follow the recommendations for reducing toxins from Day 1.

Emotional health: follow the emotional health recommendations from the morning of Day 1.

Breakfast

five-grain porridge with two tablespoons of protein powder added after cooking strawberries

Supplements: serve each child a half teaspoon of a children's probiotic powder in water or juice.

Lunch

During lunch, have everyone drink four to eight ounces of water.

green salad with mixed greens, raw goat cheese, avocado, carrots, cucumbers, celery, tomatoes, red cabbage, red peppers, red onions, and sprouts with three ounces of cold, poached, or canned wild-caught salmon (feel free to eliminate vegetables like cabbage, peppers, and onions if your children won't eat them at this time)

salad dressing: extra virgin olive oil, apple cider vinegar or lemon juice, Celtic Sea Salt, herbs, and spices; or, mix one tablespoon of extra virgin olive oil with one tablespoon of a healthy store-bought dressing

one piece of fruit in season

Dinner

During dinner, have everyone drink four to eight ounces of water.

red meat of choice

baked sweet potato with butter

steamed broccoli

green salad with mixed greens, carrots, cucumbers, celery, tomatoes, red cabbage, red peppers, red onions, and sprouts (feel free to eliminate vegetables like cabbage, peppers, and onions if your children won't eat them at this time)

salad dressing: extra virgin olive oil, apple cider vinegar or lemon juice, Celtic Sea Salt, herbs, and spices; or, mix one tablespoon of extra virgin olive oil with one tablespoon of a healthy store-bought dressing

Supplements: serve your children one or two teaspoons of a high omega-3 cod liver oil complex.

Snacks

Have everyone drink four to twelve ounces of water.

flax crackers, whole grain crackers, or baked corn chips and hummus, salsa, or guacamole one half of a berry antioxidant whole food nutrition bar with beta-glucans from soluble oat fiber

Before Bed

Have everyone drink four to eight ounces of water.

Exercise: go for a walk outdoors with your children or participate in a favorite sport or recreational activity.

Advanced hygiene: follow the advanced hygiene recommendations from the morning of Day 1.

Body therapy: give the kids a warm bath for fifteen minutes with eight drops of biblical essential oils added.

Prayer: thank God for this day, asking Him to give your children a restoring night's rest and a fresh start tomorrow. Thank Him for His steadfast love that never ceases and His mercies that are new every morning. Read 1 Corinthians 13:4–8 aloud.

Sleep: get everyone to bed fifteen minutes earlier than usual, or thirty minutes earlier if your children are still sleep deprived.

Day 8 and Beyond

If you and your children have benefited from the Great Physician's Rx for Children's Health Seven-Day Plan, you can continue to repeat the principles each week for as many times as you'd like. For more detailed step-by-step suggestions and meal and lifestyle plans, visit www.BiblicalHealthInstitute.com to find the Great Physician's Rx 49-Day Health Plan. Or, if you want to maintain your newfound level of health, you may be interested in the Lifetime of Wellness plan, which is also found on our Web site. These online programs will provide you with customized daily meal-and-exercise plans and the tools to track your family's progress.

If you've experienced positive results from the Great Physician's Rx for Children's Health program, I encourage you to reach out to someone you know and recommend this book and Seven-Day Plan to them. You can learn how to lead a small group at your church or home by visiting www.BiblicalHealthInstitute.com.

Remember, you don't have to be a pediatrician like Dr. Blair or a health expert to help transform the lives of your children—you just have to be willing.

THE GPRx
RESOURCE GUIDE

This resource section contains contact information for manufacturers and distributors of products that I recommend for parents and their children.

To the best of my ability, I am suggesting well-established companies whose health goals match mine. While I can vouch for these foods, supplements, and products, neither I nor the publisher can guarantee that these companies subscribe to the same belief system as I do, nor can we be held responsible for any possible consequences relating to the eating or ingestion of foods and/or supplements. A more complete general disclaimer is printed on the copyright page for this health-related book.

You will note that I recommend products from Garden of Life. In the interest of full disclosure, I founded this company following my illness when I had trouble finding the nutritional supplements and superfoods that my body needed. Using my knowledge gained from years of studying health and wellness, I set out to create high-quality functional foods, nutritional supplements, and educational resources to help you on your road to optimal health.

I believe that no matter which company you choose to purchase from, you will be well served on your road to vibrant health. Keep in mind that if you don't find these foods, supplements, or products in your local supermarket, natural food store, or vitamin store, you can purchase them by mail order or through online merchants. Also, if you have any questions, many of these companies can be reached via e-mail, usually through the company's Web site or by typing "info@" plus the company's Web site (example: info@gardenoflife.com).

KEY #1: TEACH THEM
TO EAT TO LIVE

Breads and Other Grain Products

Food for Life Baking Co.
P. O. Box 1434
Corona, CA 92878
(800) 797-5090
www.foodforlife.com

Food for Life, makers of Ezekiel 4:9 breads, English muffins, and tortillas, is my favorite supplier of grain products. Easily digestible, well tolerated by many who suffer from digestive ailments and allergies, and high in protein and fiber, Food for Life products truly provide the bread of life.

French Meadow Bakery
2610 Lyndale Avenue South
Minneapolis, MN 55408
(877) NO-YEAST (669-3278)
www.frenchmeadow.com

Food for Life and French Meadow products are found in natural food stores and grocery stores nationwide.

Food Bars

Living Foods Nutrition Bars by Garden of Life
(800) 622-8986
www.gardenoflife.com

Living Foods Nutrition Bars are made with organic foods such as sprouted grains and seeds, raw honey, dates, cultured vegetables, nuts, berries, green foods, and coconut. Living Foods Nutrition Bars contain beta glucans from soluble oat fiber, high-quality protein, live probiotics, antioxidants, and more.

Living Foods Nutrition Bars are great for all ages and support overall health by supporting healthy serum cholesterol and triglycerides, promoting maintenance of healthy blood sugar levels, supporting healthy immune function, and aiding in maintenance of healthy body weight.

These bars are available in health food stores nationwide, or via mail order by calling the toll-free number, or online at the Web address listed above.

Dairy Products

The following companies produce natural and organic milk, butter, cheese, cream, cottage cheese, yogurt, kefir, soft cheese, and buttermilk that are either available in natural food stores or by mail order.

Old Chatham Sheepherding Company
155 Shaker Museum Road
Old Chatham, NY 12136
(888) SHEEP-60 (743-3760)
www.blacksheepcheese.com

Old Chatham makes the finest quality sheep's milk yogurt and cheese. This is the yogurt our family eats and Joshua's favorite. It is available via mail order or in select natural food stores.

Amaltheia Dairy
3380 Penwell Bridge Road
Belgrade, MT 59714
(406) 388-5950
www.amaltheiadairy.com

Grade A goat's dairy kefir and cheeses. Available via mail order and in select natural food stores.

Organic Pastures Dairy Co.
7221 South Jameson Avenue
Fresno, CA 93706
(877) RAW-MILK (729-6455)
www.organicpastures.com

Coconut Milk

Thai Kitchen Coconut Milk
Epicurean International, Inc.
30315 Union City Blvd.
Union City, CA 94587
(800) 967-8424
www.thaikitchen.com

Thai Kitchen products are available in natural food stores nationwide.

Eggs

Gold Circle Farms
310 N. Harbor Blvd., Suite 205
Fullerton, CA 92832
(888) 599-4DHA (4342)
www.goldcirclefarms.com

These DHA omega-3 eggs are available in natural food stores and grocery stores nationwide.

Organic Valley
One Organic Way
La Farge, WI 54639
(888) 444-6455
www.organicvalley.com

These certified organic high omega-3 eggs are available in natural food stores and grocery stores nationwide.

Red Meats

Real Foods Market
743 West 1200 North, Suite 200
Springville, UT 84663
(866) 284-7325
www.realfoodsmarket.com

Wyoming Natural Products Co.
P. O. Box 962
Newcastle, WY 82701
(800) 969-9946
www.wyomingnatural.com
Their grass-fed beef is available in select natural food stores and via mail order.

Maverick Ranch Natural Meats
5360 North Franklin Street
Denver, CO 80216
(800) 497-2624
www.maverickranch.com
This natural beef, chicken, lamb, and buffalo is available in grocery stores nationwide.

Coleman Purely Natural Products
1767 Denver West Marriott Blvd., Suite 200
Golden, CO 80401
(800) 442-8666
www.colemannatural.com
These naturally raised, hormone- and antibiotic-free beef products are available in natural food stores nationwide.

Northstar Bison
1936 28th Ave.
Rice Lake, WI 54868
(888) 295-6332
www.northstarbison.com
They supply one hundred percent grass-fed and finished bison meat.

Chicken

Oaklyn Plantation
1312 Oaklyn Road
Darlington, SC 29532
(843) 395-0793
www.freerangechicken.com
These free-range chickens and chicken feet (hormone- and antibiotic-free) are available via mail order.

Bell & Evans
154 W. Main St.
Fredericksburg, PA 17026
(717) 865-6626
www.bellandevans.com

These fresh and frozen natural poultry products are available in natural food stores and grocery stores nationwide.

Deli Meat

Applegate Farms
750 Rt. 202 South, 3rd Floor
Bridgewater, NJ 08807
(800) 587-5858
www.applegatefarms.com

These packaged meats and deli slices (nitrate- and nitrite-free) are available in natural food stores and grocery stores nationwide.

Frozen Fish

Ecofish
340 Central Ave.
Dover, NH 03820
(877) 214-3474
www.ecofish.com

Their ocean-caught salmon, halibut, tuna, and other fish are available in natural food stores and grocery stores nationwide.

Vital Choice Seafood
P. O. Box 4121
Bellingham, WA 98227
(800) 608-4825
www.vitalchoice.com

Their products are available in natural food stores nationwide.

Crown Prince
18581 Railroad Street
City of Industry, CA 91748
(800) 255-5063
www.crownprince.com

These canned sardines, salmon, tuna, and other fish are available in natural food stores and grocery stores nationwide.

Honey

Hawaiian Lehua Honey by Garden of Life
(800) 622-8986
www.gardenoflife.com

This certified organic honey comes from the island of Hawaii. Hawaiian Lehua Honey contains antioxidants, enzymes, vitamins, and minerals, providing all of the benefits that make honey a superfood from the hive. This raw, unheated honey is the original sweetener used for thousands of years and is a superb resource to sweeten smoothies, yogurt, tea, and coffee. This honey is also an important ingredient in many of the delicious recipes you'll find in this book.

It is available via mail order by calling the toll-free number, or online at the Web address listed above.

Sweeteners

Rapadura Whole Cane Sugar
Global Organic Brands
37 West 20th Street, Suite 708
New York, NY 10011
(800) 207-2814
www.rapunzel.com

Salad Mixes (prewashed)

Earthbound Farm
1721 San Juan Highway
San Juan Bautista, CA 95045
(800) 690-3200
www.ebfarm.com

This fresh, packaged organic produce is available in natural food stores and grocery stores nationwide.

Vegetables (including raw fermented)

Earthbound Farm
1721 San Juan Highway
San Juan Bautista, CA 95045
(800) 690-3200
www.ebfarm.com

This fresh, organic produce is available in natural food stories and grocery stores nationwide.

Rejuvenative Foods
P. O. Box 8464
Santa Cruz, CA 95061
(800) 805-7957
www.rejuvenative.com

Rejuvenative Foods produces high-quality raw foods such as sauerkraut, kimchi, "live" salsas, nut and seed butters, chocolate spreads, raw oils, and more. These products are available in some grocery and health food stores, and online via mail order.

Frozen Fruits and Vegetables

Cascadian Farms
Small Planet Foods
P. O. Box 9452
Minneapolis, MN 55440
(800) 624-4123
www.cfarm.com

These frozen, packaged organic fruits and vegetables, including berries, are available in health food and grocery stores nationwide.

Protein Powder (from goat's milk)

Goatein by Garden of Life
(800) 622-8986
www.gardenoflife.com

Goatein, an exceptional goat's milk protein powder, is a source of eight essential amino acids crucial to good health. Easy to digest, Goatein is well tolerated by those who cannot digest cow's milk and is available in natural food stores, from mail-order catalogs, and through online retailers nationwide.

Extra Virgin Coconut Oil

Garden of Life
(800) 622-8986
www.gardenoflife.com

Once thought to be a "bad" fat, coconut oil has been shown to be a stable, healthy saturated fat. In fact, extra virgin coconut oil is one of the healthiest and most versatile unprocessed dietary oils in the world. Garden of Life Extra Virgin Coconut Oil is an unprocessed culinary oil full of natural coconut flavor and aroma. It is available in natural food stores, from mail-order catalogs, and through online retailers nationwide.

Apple Cider, Organic Balsamic, or Other Vinegars

Bragg Live Foods
P. O. Box 7
Santa Barbara, CA 93102
(800) 446-1990
www.bragg.com

This apple cider vinegar made from organically grown apples, as well as other natural products, is available in health food and grocery stores nationwide.

Nuts and Seeds

Living Nutz
P. O. Box 11413
Portland, ME 04104
(207) 780-1101
www.livingnutz.com

Their variety of low-temperature-dried sprouted nuts are available in select natural food stores and via mail order.

Nut and Seed Butters

Rejuvenative Foods
P. O. Box 8464
Santa Cruz, CA 95061
(800) 805-7957
www.rejuvenative.com

These highest-quality, best-tasting raw organic nut and seed butters—including those made from almond, sesame, pumpkin, cashew, and sunflower seeds—are available in some grocery and health food stores, by mail order, or through online merchants.

Tea

Living Tea by Garden of Life
(800) 622-8986
www.gardenoflife.com

These certified organic green, black, and rooibos teas are delivered in convenient liquid-packs. Wellness Tea is great as hot or iced tea and comes in many flavors: unflavored green tea, raspberry green tea, lemon green tea, peach green tea, and coffee-flavored black and rooibos tea. Wellness Tea is loaded with antioxidants and the exciting compound epigallocatechin gallate, or EGCG.

These teas are available with or without caffeine, from natural food stores and via mail-order catalogs and online retailers nationwide.

Sea Salt

Celtic Sea Salt
Grain & Salt Society
Four Celtic Drive
Arden, NC 28704
(800) 867-7258
www.celticseasalt.com

Celtic Sea Salt (coarse and fine) is available in some health food stores and grocery stores.

RealSalt
P. O. Box 219
Redmond, UT 84652
(800) FOR-SALT (367-7258)
www.realsalt.com

RealSalt is mined in central Utah, and is available in health food and grocery stores.

Organic Spices

Simply Organic
Frontier Natural Products
P. O. Box 299
Norway, IA 52318
(800) 669-3275
www.frontiercoop.com

These are packaged organic spices in glass jars.

Condiments

Spectrum Organic Products
5341 Old Redwood Highway,
Suite 400
Petaluma, CA 94954
(800) 995-2705
www.spectrumorganics.com

This healthy, organic, omega-3 mayonnaise uses expeller-pressed soy and flaxseed oils, and is available in some health food stores and grocery stores.

Westbrae Natural Foods
Novelco Distribution
P. O. Box 1346
Downey, CA 90240
(562) 215-4843
www.novelco.com/westbrae

This natural ketchup and mustard is available in some health food stores and grocery stores.

Flaxseed Oil

Barlean's Organic Oils
4936 Lake Terrell Road
Ferndale, WA 98248
(360) 384-0485
www.barleans.com

Their organic high-lignan flaxseed oil and borage seed oil, as well as flaxseed fiber is available at health food stores nationwide.

Organic Vegetable Oils

Garden of Life
(800) 622-8986
www.gardenoflife.com

These are high-quality organic oils, including extra virgin olive oil.

Bionaturae
5 Tyler Drive
North Franklin, CT 06254
(860) 642-6996
www.bionaturae.com

They supply organic extra virgin olive oil.

Raw Almond Oil, Evening Primrose Oil, Sunflower Oil, and Poppy Seed Oil

Raw Oils from Rejuvenative Foods
P. O. Box 8464
Santa Cruz, CA 95061
(800) 805-7957
www.rawoils.com

Extra Virgin Olive Oil

Bariani Olive Oil
1330 Waller Street
San Francisco, CA 94117
(415) 864-1917
www.barianioliveoil.com

Organic Chocolate Spreads

Rejuvenative Foods
P. O. Box 8464
Santa Cruz, CA 95061
(800) 805-7957
www.rejuvenative.com

These healthy organic chocolate spreads are great for all ages.

Flaxseed Crackers

Glaser Organic Farms
19100 SW 137th Avenue
Miami, FL 33012
(305) 238-7747
www.glaserorganicfarms.com

Food Preparation/Utensils

Mercola.com
www.mercola.com

These food preparation tools, such as juicers and convection ovens, are available online.

Vita-Mix Blender
8615 Usher Road
Cleveland, OH 44138
(800) 848-2649
www.vitamix.com

Their high-quality, durable blender is excellent for smoothies and soups—a must-have for every health-conscious family.

For more information on eating to live, visit www.BiblicalHealth Institute.com.

KEY #2: SUPPLEMENT THEIR DIETS WITH WHOLE FOOD NUTRITIONAL SUPPLEMENTS

Whole Food Multivitamins (with zinc)

Living Multi by Garden of Life
(800) 622-8986
www.gardenoflife.com

Living Multi is a complete vitamin and mineral supplement that delivers superfoods to support your demanding nutritional needs. This comprehensive whole food multinutrient formula contains fruits, vegetables, ocean plants, tonic mushrooms, botanicals, and ionic minerals including enzymes, antioxidants, amino acids, and homeostatic nutrient complexes. Living Multi is available in natural food stores, from mail-order catalogs, and through online retailers nationwide.

Daily Foundation Pack by Trivita
(800) 991-7116
www.trivita.com

The daily foundation pack by Trivita is a three-product combination containing vitamins and minerals, including sublingual B-12, B-6, folic acid and Vitamin C.

Women's Wellness Daily by Silver Creek Laboratories
(800) 493-1146
www.silvercreeklabs.com

This multivitamin/mineral formula is designed specifically for a woman's needs.

Botanical Immune Support Blend with Garlic, Ginger, Elderberry, and Echinacea

Seasonal Relief by Garden of Life
(800) 622-8986
www.gardenoflife.com

Seasonal Relief is a botanical blend of immune supportive herbs and spices that have been used for thousands of years.

Wellness Formula by Source Naturals
www.sourcenaturals.com

Esberitox by Enzymatic Therapy
(800) 783-2286
www.enzy.com

Botanical Essential Oil and CO2 Extract Liquicap Blends

Alpha AM Cleanse and Omega
PM Cleanse
by Garden of Life
(866) 985-GPRX
www.GreatPhysiciansRx.com

These are blends of essential oils and CO_2 extracts from herbs and spices that were used in biblical times to support immune system health and provide a concentrated source of antioxidants.

Oil of Oregano by Gaia Herbs
(828) 884-4242
www.gaiaherbs.com

This high-quality extract of oregano has been used for centuries to aid in respiratory and immune system health.

Immune Support
Echinacea-Ginger Tonic
www.new-chapter.com

Omega-3 Cod Liver Oil

Olde World Icelandic Cod Liver Oil
by Garden of Life
(800) 622-8986
www.gardenoflife.com

Olde World Icelandic Cod Liver Oil is one of nature's richest sources of vitamins A and D, which can play an important role in supporting cardio-vascular health. To ensure that its naturally occurring ingredients remain intact, Olde World Icelandic Cod Liver Oil is always harvested from the pure cold waters of Iceland and is cold-processed using traditional methods. Olde World Icelandic Cod Liver Oil is available in natural food stores, from mail-order catalogs, and through online merchants nationwide.

Fresh Catch Fish Oil
by Ribbon Nutrition
(800) 757-7212
www.ribbonnutrition.com

This is an excellent fish oil product with EPA and DHA.

Green Food/Fiber Blend

Perfect Food by Garden of Life
(800) 622-8986
www.gardenoflife.com

Perfect Food is a green superfood containing organic ingredients, including cereal grass juices, micro-algaes, vegetable juice concentrates, sprouts, and seeds. Perfect Food provides antioxidants, enzymes, chlorophyll, and trace minerals, and is available in natural food stores and through online retailers.

SuperSeed by Garden of Life
(800) 622-8986
www.gardenoflife.com

SuperSeed is a whole food fiber blend containing organic ingredients including sprouted and fermented seeds, grains, and legumes. SuperSeed is available in natural food stores, from mail-order catalogs, and through online retailers nationwide.

Green Food Complex by Trivita
(800) 991-7116
www.trivita.com

This superb green superfood comes in both powder and capsules and contains the juice of young barley and alfalfa grasses.

Probiotics and Enzymes

Primal Defense Kid's by Garden of Life
(800) 622-8986
www.gardenoflife.com

Primal Defense Kid's contains probiotics and prebiotics in a delicious-tasting banana flavor. This whole food probiotic blend promotes overall wellness and is available in natural food stores, from mail-order catalogs, and through online retailers nationwide.

Omega Zyme by Garden of Life
(800) 622-8986
www.gardenoflife.com

Omega Zyme is a whole food digestive enzyme blend that supports gastrointestinal health, carbohydrate digestion, and normal bowel function. It is available in natural food stores, from mail-order catalogs, and through online retailers.

Digestive Complex by Trivita
(800) 991-7116
www.trivita.com

This digestive formula contains enzymes and probiotics to support digestion and elimination.

Antioxidant/Energy Formula with B Vitamins, Folic Acid, and Chromium

Clear Energy by Garden of Life
(800) 622-8986
www.gardenoflife.com

Clear Energy is designed to support overall health and wellness, manage stress and promote energy, and promote stamina and mental clarity as well as concentration. Clear Energy contains whole food B vitamins to support healthy cardiovascular function, herbal adaptogens to manage stress, and extracts from beverages to promote cellular energy.

Core Antioxidant
by Ribbon Nutrition
(800) 757-7212
www.ribbonnutrition.com
This is a high quality botanical antioxidant and energy formula.

KEY #3: INTRODUCE YOUR CHILDREN TO ADVANCED HYGIENE

Advanced Hygiene Products

Advanced Hygiene System
by Garden of Life
(800) 622-8986
www.gardenoflife.com
Advanced Hygiene System supports vibrant health by thoroughly cleansing the areas of your body most vulnerable to germs: hands, eyes, mouth, ears, and nose. This advanced hygiene product reinforces overall health and well-being, promotes clear skin, and refreshes teeth and gums. Call the toll-free number or visit the Web site for more information.

Bausch & Lomb
One Bausch & Lomb Place
Rochester, NY 14604-2701
(585) 338-6000
www.bausch.com
Bausch & Lomb Eye Wash and Eye Irrigating Solution flushes away foreign objects, chlorine, and other eye irritants, and is available in supermarkets and drugstores nationwide.

Xlear
P. O. Box 970911
Orem, UT 84097
(877) 599-5327
www.xlear.com
This all natural, drug-free nasal wash is available in natural food stores nationwide.

Clay Neti Pots by the Planet
5111-A NW 13th St.
Gainesville, FL 32609
(888) 543-9294
www.bytheplanet.com
This product is helpful in relieving sinus and nasal passage congestion.

For more information on practicing advanced hygiene, visit www.BiblicalHealthInstitute.com.

KEY #4: CONDITION THEIR BODIES
WITH EXERCISE AND BODY
THERAPIES

Aromatherapy with Essential Oils

AlphaAromaTherapy and Omega Aroma Therapy by Garden of Life
(866) 985-GPRX
www.GreatPhysiciansRx.com

These are blends of essential oils and CO_2 extracts from herbs and spices used extensively in biblical times. These products are great for use in therapeutic baths.

Oshadhi
1340-G Industrial Ave.
Petaluma, CA 94952
(888) OSHADHI (674-2344)
www.oshadhiusa.com

They supply undiluted organic essential oils.

Functional Fitness Video

Functional Fitness DVD
by Garden of Life
(800) 622-8986
www.gardenoflife.com

Experience the energizing, enjoyable world of functional fitness exercise. Functional exercise teaches you to train whole body movements, not just isolated muscles, increasing fitness, coordination, flexibility, and agility while decreasing your chances of injury during daily activity. Featuring fun and easy routines that can be performed anywhere and anytime, functional fitness is great for people of any age or skill level. Call the toll-free number or visit the Web site for more information.

Rebounders

Optimum Performance Systems
438 NW 13th Street
Boca Raton, Florida, 33432
(561) 393-3881
www.opsfit.com

This is an excellent resource for exercise videos, books, and programs for recreational, amateur, and professional athletes.

Rebound Air
993 North 450 West
Springville, UT 84663
(888) 464-JUMP (5867)
www.reboundair.com

This is a supplier of rebounders, great for low-impact exercise.

Lympholine
Life Source International
1112 Montana Ave., Suite 125
Santa Monica, CA 90403
(310) 284-3565
www.lympholine.com

The Lympholine rebounder activates the lymphatic system to purify the body.

Needak Manufacturing
P.O. Box 776
O'Neill, NE 68763
(800) 232-5762
www.needak-rebounders.com

For more information on conditioning your body with exercise and body therapies, visit www.Biblical HealthInstitute.com.

KEY #5: REDUCE TOXINS IN THEIR
ENVIRONMENTS

Skin and Body Care

Organic Skin Systems
by Garden of Life
(800) 622-8986
www.gardenoflife.com

Organic Skin Systems is the first skin and body care line using probiotics, whole food vitamins, minerals, and antioxidants. Organic Skin Systems is free of chemicals and is designed to promote healthy skin for the entire body.

Aubrey Organics
4419 N. Manhattan Ave.
Tampa, FL 33614
(813) 877-4186
www.aubrey-organics.com

Aubrey Hampton, the founder of Aubrey Organics, has been formulating and manufacturing skin and body care products for thirty years. Aubrey produces hundreds of products, including skin care, hair care, soaps and cleansers, toothpaste, natural hair color, and perfumes and colognes.

MyChelle Dermaceuticals
P. O. Box 1
Frisco, CO 80443
(800) 447-2076
www.mychelleusa.com

MyChelle Dermaceuticals utilizes innovative fruit, vegetables, and enzymes in their products to deliver outstanding results for men and women.

Miracle Distributors
P. O. Box 2455
Matthews, NC 28106
(866) 567-2326
www.miracledistributors.com

Nontoxic soaps and cleansers great for hair, skin, and home.

*Extra Virgin Coconut Oil
by Garden of Life*
(800) 622-8986
www.gardenoflife.com

Coconut oil has been traditionally used by tropical cultures to condition skin during and after sun exposure. It is available in natural food stores and through online retailers.

Cosmetics

Peacekeeper Cosmetics
350 Third Avenue #351
New York, NY 10010
(866) 732-2336
www.iamapeacekeeper.com

In addition to quality ingredients, the company donates all profits, after taxes, to support women's health advocacy and human rights issues.

Cleaning Supplies
---

*PerfectClean Ultramicrofiber
Mops, Wipes, and Dusters*
www.SixWise.com

Indoor pollution has become one of the leading causes of disease. A main health risk is dust, which commonly contains over twenty toxins, such as heavy metals, PCBs, viruses, bacteria, and allergens. I urge you to throw away your typical mops, sponges, and wipers, which do a remarkably poor job of eliminating dust and biological contaminants. These products also require the use of chemical cleaners, which only introduce more toxins into your environment.

Instead, I recommend the Perfect-Clean line of mops, wipes, and dusters, which are available exclusively at one of my favorite Web sites, www.SixWise.com. PerfectClean's innovative "ultramicrober" construction means that with just the use of water—no chemical cleaners required—the surfaces in your home will become clean down to the microscopic level, eliminating even the biological contaminants that no other cleaning tool or solution can touch. PerfectClean lasts for hundreds of uses, so it's also economical.

PerfectClean products can be found online at www.SixWise.com.

Bi-O-Kleen
P. O. Box 820689
Vancouver, WA 98682
(800) 477-0188
www.bi-o-kleen.com
Try Turbo Plus Ceramic Laundry Discs and Flora Brite papaya enzyme laundry additive and whitener.

Orange TKO
3395 S. Jones Blvd. #221
Las Vegas, NV 89146
(800) 995-2463
www.tkoorange.com
This is an all-purpose cleaner, stain remover, and odor remover made from organic orange oil.

Seventh Generation
212 Battery St., Suite A
Burlington, VT 05401
(800) 456-1191
www.seventhgeneration.com

Air Purifiers

Pionair
813 Pavilion Ct.
McDonough, GA 30253
(866) PIONAIR (746-6247)
www.pionair.net
The Pionair air purification system enhances the quality of air in the home and reduces harmful toxins such as yeasts, molds, bacteria, and debris. It is available in select health stores and via mail order.

Water Purifiers

New Wave Enviro Products
P. O. Box 4146
Englewood, CO 80155
(800) 592-8371
www.newwaveenviro.com
These water purifiers and shower filters remove harmful toxins, including chlorine.

Produce Wash

Veggie Wash
Beaumont Products
1560 Big Shanty Dr.
Kennesaw, GA 30144
(800) 451-7096
www.citrusmagic.com

Made with 100 percent natural ingredients derived from citrus fruit, corn, and coconut, Veggie Wash aids in the removal of pesticides, germs, and toxins from fruits and produce.

Paper Products

Seventh Generation
212 Battery Street, Suite A
Burlington, VT 05401
(800) 456-1191
www.seventhgeneration.com

They supply unbleached paper towels, napkins, toilet paper, and tissue.

Feminine Products

Organic Essentials
822 Baldridge St.
O'Donnell, TX 79351
(800) 765-6491
www.organicessentials.com

Organic Essentials also produces organic cotton balls and cotton swabs.

Organic Clothing

Under the Canopy
3601 North Dixie Hwy., Bay 1
Boca Raton, FL 33431
(888) 226-6799
www.underthecanopy.com

They are the world's largest source of modern and sophisticated organic fiber fashions for women, men, and children.

Nontoxic Carpeting and Other Building Materials

Building for Health
P. O. Box 113
Carbondale, CO 81623
(800) 292-4838
www.buildingforhealth.com

This is a resource for nontoxic carpets and other nontoxic building materials.

For more information on reducing toxins in your environment, visit www.BiblicalHealth Institute.com.

Key #6: Help Them Avoid Deadly Emotions

For more information on avoiding deadly emotions, visit www.Biblical HealthInstitute.com.

Key #7: Lead Them to Live Lives of Prayer and Purpose

For more information on living a life of prayer and purpose, visit www.BiblicalHealthInstitute.com.

ABOUT THE AUTHORS

Jordan Rubin has dedicated his life to transforming the health of God's people one life at a time. He is the founder and chairman of the Biblical Health Institute, an organization dedicated to providing biblical health education and resources, and Garden of Life, Inc., a health and wellness company based in West Palm Beach, Florida, that produces organic functional foods, whole food nutritional supplements, and personal care products. Jordan frequently ministers in churches and at Christian conferences worldwide to tens of thousands of people each year.

He and his wife, Nicki, are the parents of a three-year-old son, Joshua. They make their home in Palm Beach Gardens, Florida.

Fiona Blair, M.D., a Harvard University graduate who earned a medical degree at Emory University, is a board-certified pediatrician in the Atlanta area. She has appeared numerous times on *CNN Headline News* as a medical expert whenever the topic of childhood obesity has made the news. A mother of four, Dr. Blair, and her husband, Everton, make their home in Stone Mountain, Georgia.

NOTES

Introduction

1. A *doula* is a woman experienced in childbirth who provides emotional support and physical comfort during the birthing process.

2. Chris Niles, "Tart Emeritus: Miss Piggy," Tart City, http://www.tartcity.com/misspiggy.html (accessed June 18, 2007).

3. Sally Squires, "The Heavy Burden of Stereotyping," *Washington Post*, May 9, 2006, HE1.

4. Ibid.

5. *Progress in Preventing Childhood Obesity: How Do We Measure Up?*, National Academies Press, 2006. This report is available at http://www.nap.edu/catalog/11722.html#toc (accessed June 18, 2007).

6. Rick Reilly, "The Fat of the Land," *Sports Illustrated*, September 16, 2003, http://palosverdeshigh.net/My_web/myweb/child%20obesity%20art.htm (accessed June 18, 2007).

7. Ibid.

8. "Obesity in Youth" fact sheet from the American Obesity Association, available at http://obesityusa.org/subs/fastfacts/obesity_youth.shtml (accessed June 18, 2007).

9. Calum MacLeod, "Obesity of China's Kids Stuns Officials," *USA Today*, January 9, 2007.

10. "Overweight in Early Childhood Increases Chances for Obesity at Age 12," a National Institutes of Health press release issued September 5, 2006, and available at http://www.nih.gov/news/pr/sep2006/nichd-05.htm (accessed June 18, 2007).

11. Theresa Agovino, "Prescriptions Treating or Preventing Type 2 Diabetes in Children Doubles in Four Years," Associated Press, April 4, 2006.

12. Jeffrey Krasner, "Diabetes Therapy Deal," *Boston Globe*, March 16, 2005, http://www.iht.com/articles/2005/03/15/business/genzyme.php (accessed June 18, 2007).

13. "Deaths: Preliminary Data for 2004," National Center for Health Statistics, available online at http://www.cdc.gov/nchs/data/hestat/preliminarydeaths04_tables.pdf (accessed June 18, 2007).

14. David S. Freedman et al., "The Relation of Overweight to Cardiovascular Risk Factors Among Children and Adolescents: The Bogalusa Heart Study," *Journal of Pediatrics* 103, no. 6 (1999): 1175–82.

15. William H. Dietz, "Health Consequences of Obesity in Youth: Childhood Predictors of Adult Disease," *Pediatriatrics* 101, no. 3 supplement (March 1998): 518–25, http://pediatrics.aappublications.org/cgi/content/abstract/101/3/S1/518 (accessed June 18, 2007).

16. Associated Press, "Overweight Children Are More at Risk for Broken Bones and Joint Problems," November 22, 2005, http://health.usnews.com/usnews/health/briefs/childrenshealth/hb051122a.htm (accessed June 18, 2007).

17. Reilly, "The Fat of the Land."

18. James A. Fowler, "Some Thoughts on Parenting," Christ in You Ministries Web site, http://www.christinyou.net/pages/thotsparent.html (accessed June 18, 2007).

19. Ibid.

20. Gina Kolata, "So Big and Healthy Grandpa Wouldn't Even Know You," *New York Times*, July 30, 2006, http://www.iht.com/articles/2006/07/30/healthscience/web.0730age.php (accessed June 18, 2007).

21. Kathleen Doheny, "Strict Parenting Can Produce Overweight Kids," *HealthDay* online magazine, June 6, 2006, and available at http://www.forbes.com/forbeslife/health/feeds/hscout/2006/06/06/hscout533082.html (accessed June 18, 2007).

22. Peter Salgo, "The Doctor Will See You in Exactly Seven Minutes," The New York Times, March 22, 2006, http://www.nytimes.com/2006/03/22/opinion/22salgo.html?ex=1300683600&en=d699ad96f30ac4c0&ei=5088&partner=rssnyt&emc=rss (accessed July 20, 2007).

Key #1

1. Bill Gibron, "Simple Rules," *PopMatters*, April 27, 2006, http://www.popmatters.com/tv/reviews/h/honey-were-killing-the-kids-060427.shtml (accessed June 18, 2007).

2. "Lifestyle and Obesity: How Occasional Indulgences Shape a Nation's Waistline," a Thomson Medstat Research Brief, July 2006, http://www.medstat.com/uploadedFiles/docs/Research%20Brief--Lifestyle%20and%20Obesity.pdf (accessed June 18, 2007).

3. Eric Schlosser, *Fast Food Nation* (New York: Houghton Mifflin, 2001), 10.

4. Caroline E. Mayer, "TV Ads Entice Kids to Overeat, Study Finds," *Washington Post*, December 7, 2005, D1, http://www.washingtonpost.com/wp-dyn/content/ article/2005/12/06/AR2005120600671.html (accessed June 18, 2007).

5. Susan M. Connor, "Food-Related Advertising on Preschool Television: Building Brand Recognition in Young Viewers," *Pediatrics* 118, no. 4 (October 2006): 1478–85, http://pediatrics.aappublications.org/cgi/content/abstract/118/4/1478 (accessed June 18, 2007).

6. "Role of TV Ads in Kids' Obesity? FCC to Study," Associated Press, September 27, 2006, http://www.msnbc.msn.com/id/15035381/ (accessed June 18, 2007).

7. Patrick Goldstein, "Studios Feast on Fast-Food Tie-Ins," *Los Angeles Times*, November 21, 2006, E1.

8. Gina Bellafante, "An Athlete Who Puts It All on the Table," *New York Times*, January 18, 2006.

9. Carolyn O'Neil, "Kids Will Fill Up on Parents' Example," *Atlanta Journal-Constitution*, November 1, 2006, http://www.ajc.com/blogs/content/shared-blogs/ajc/ healthyeating/entries/2006/11/01/post_3.html (accessed June 18, 2007).

10. Elisabeth Leamy, "Secrets in Your Food," ABC News Web site, August 21, 2006, http://abcnews.go.com/GMA/story?id=2337731&page=1 (accessed June 18, 2007).

11. David Pierson, "No Shortage of Oil at the L.A. County Fair," *Los Angeles Times*, September 21, 2006, A1, http://www.latimes.com/news/local/la-me-fried21sep21,0,2647864.story?coll=la-home-headlines (accessed June 18, 2007).

12. Dr. Joseph Mercola, *Dr. Joseph Mercola's "eHealthy News You Can Use,"* December 7, 2006, issue 882 (video clip), http://www.mercola.com/2006/dec/7 (accessed June 18, 2007).

13. "4 Most Harmful Ingredients in Packaged Foods," *Reader's Digest* Web site, http://www.rd.com/content/4-most-harmful-ingredients-in-packaged-foods/ (accessed June 18, 2007).

14. "Manic for Organic," *Los Angeles Times* (editorial), March 10, 2006, B12, http://ofrf.org/pressroom/organic_news_clips/060310_latimes_oped_manicfororganic.pdf (accessed June 18, 2007).

15. Kathleen Kiley, "Private Label Meets Organic Food," *KPMG Consumer Markets Insider*, October 6, 2006; and Parija Bhatnagar, "Wal-Mart's Next Conquest: Organics," CNNMoney.com Web site, May 1, 2006, http://money.cnn.com/2006/05/01/news/ companies/walmart_organics/ (accessed June 19, 2007).

16. Melanie Warner, "Wal-Mart Eyes Organic Foods," *New York Times*, May 12, 2006, http://www.nytimes.com/2006/05/12/business/12organic.html?ex=1305086400en=b8ee 8ab04d4a6d72ei=5088partner=rssnytemc=rss (accessed June 19, 2007).

17. "Cutting Trans Fats," *San Diego Union-Tribune* editorial, December 21, 2006, B6, http://www.signonsandiego.com/uniontrib/20061221/news_lz1ed21bottom.html (accessed June 19, 2007).

18. Susan Perry, "Fat Chance," *Lifetime Fitness* magazine, January/February 2006 issue, http://www.lifetimefitness.com/magazine/index.cfm?strWebAction=article_detail&intArti cleId=498 (accessed June 19, 2007).

19. Libby Quaid, "Poll: Overweight America Does Read Labels," Associated Press, July 2, 2006. Article available online at http://www.cbsnews.com/stories/2006/07/02/ap/health/mainD8IJV0KO0.shtml (accessed June 19, 2007).

20. Jerry Hirsch, "Lawsuit Stirs Up Guacamole Labeling Controversy," *Los Angeles Times*, November 30, 2006, C1, available online at http://soundingcircle.com/newslog2.php /__show_article/_a000195-001084.htm (accessed June 19, 2007).

21. Nina Planck, "Death by Veganism," *New York Times*, May 21, 2007, http://www.nytimes.com/2007/05/21/opinion/21planck.html?ex=1182398400&en=110 f8185909fc3da&ei=5070 (accessed June 19, 2007).

22. "Vegetarian & Vegan Related Quotes," famousveggies.com Web site, http://www.famousveggie.com/quotes.cfm (accessed June 19, 2007).

23. Sally Fallon, *Nourishing Traditions* (Washington, DC: New Trends Publishing, Inc., 2001), 27.

24. "National Survey Reveals 80 Percent of Americans Eat Meat More Than Three Times per Week," May 9, 2006, http://www.wholefoodsmarket.com/company/pr_05-09-06.html (accessed June 19, 2007).

25. "What Are the Health Risks Associated with Factory Farms?", Grace Factory Farm Project Web site, http://factoryfarm.org/whatis/2.php (accessed June 19, 2007).

26. Daniel DeNoon, "Salt-Water Fish Extinction Seen by 2048," WebMD, November 3, 2006, http://www.cbsnews.com/stories/2006/11/02/health/webmd/main2147223.shtml (accessed June 19, 2007).

27. Sally Fallon with Mary G. Enig, Ph.D., *Nourishing Traditions: The Cookbook That Challenges Politically Correct Nutrition and the Diet Dictocrats* (Washington, D.C.: NewTrends Publishing, 2000), 28.

28. William Campbell Douglass II, M.D., *The Milk Book: The Milk of Human Kindness Is Not Pasteurized*, 3rd ed. (Panama, Republic of Panama: Rhino Publishing, 2003), 2.

29. Andy Rooney, "What Have They Done to Milk?" commentary on CBS *60 Minutes*, June 11, 2006, available at http://www.cbsnews.com/stories/2005/11/03/60minutes/rooney/main1007432.shtml (accessed June 19, 2007).

30. Douglass, *The Milk Book*, 42.

31. J. M. Peters et al., "Processed Meats and Risk of Childhood Leukemia (California, USA)," *Cancer Causes Control* 5, no. 2 (March 1994):195–202. Abstract available online at http://www.ncbi.nlm.nih.gov/sites/entrez?cmd=Retrieve&db=PubMed&list_uids=8167267&dopt=Abstract (accessed June 19, 2007).

32. P. Samuel, et al., "Effect of Breakfast Composition on Cognitive Processes in Elementary School Children," *Physiology & Behavior* 85, no. 5 (2005): 635–45. Abstract available online at http://www.cababstractsplus.org/google/abstract.asp?AcNo=20053156975 (accessed June 19, 2007).

33. Dr. Joseph Mercola, "Where's the Fiber in Whole Grain Cereals?" Mercola.com, http://www.mercola.com/2005/feb/23/cereal_fiber.htm (accessed July 20, 2007).

34. "School Lunches," *National Geographic*, September 2006.

35. Scott Malone, "Kerfuffle over 'Fluffernutters' in Massachusetts," Reuters, June 21, 2006.

36. Nancy Gibbs, "The Magic of the Family Meal," *Time*, June 4, 2006, http://www.time.com/time/magazine/article/0,9171,1200760,00.html (accessed June 19, 2007).

37. Barbara J. Mayfield, M.S., R.D., "Family Meals Fact Sheet," available online at http://www.familymeals.org/PDFs/Family_Meals_Fact_Sheet.pdf (accessed June 19, 2007).

38. F. Batmanghelidj, M.D., *You're Not Sick, You're Thirsty!* (New York: Warner Books, 2003), 50.

39. "Chicken Soup, Rx for the Cold," Health A to Z Web site, http://www.healthatoz.com/healthatoz/Atoz/dc/caz/resp/cold/chixsoup.jsp (accessed June 19, 2007).

40. "Are There More Sheep or People in New Zealand?", About.com: site, http://geography.about.com/library/faq/blqzsheep.htm (accessed June 19, 2007).

Key #2

1. "Flintstones Children's Complete Multivitamins—We Finally Have Betty and the Great Gazoo!!", a review of Flintstones Children's Complete Multivitamins on Epinions.com, December 13, 2002, http://www1.epinions.com/content_83562827396 (accessed June 19, 2007).

2. Theresa Gallagher, "ADDers Are More Likely to Have Fatty Acid Deficiencies," http://www.mercola.com/beef/adhd.htm (accessed June 19, 2007).

3. Stephen Daniells, "Scientists Probe Omega-3 DHA as Anti-Obesity Agent," *NutraIngredients News*, November 20, 2006, http://www.nutraingredients.com/news/ng.asp?n=72168-dha-omega-anti-obesity (accessed June 20, 2007).

4. Ingrid B. Helland, M.D., et al., "Maternal Supplementation with Very-Long-Chain n-3 Fatty Acids During Pregnancy and Lactation Augments Children's IQ at 4 Years of Age," *Pediatrics* 111, no. 1 (January 2003): e39–e44, http://pediatrics.aappublications.org/cgi/content/abstract/111/1/e39 (accessed June 20, 2007).

5. John Paul SanGiovanni, et al., "Meta-analysis of Dietary Essential Fatty Acids and Long-Chain Polyunsaturated Fatty Acids as They Relate to Visual Resolution Acuity in Healthy Preterm Infants," *Pediatrics* 105, no. 6 (June 2000): 1292–98. Abstract available at http://pediatrics.aappublications.org/cgi/content/abstract/105/6/1292?ck=nck (accessed June 20, 2007).

6. Gallagher, "ADDers More Likely to Have Fatty Acid Deficiencies."

7. Krispin Sullivan, quoting David Horrobin, "Cod Liver Oil: The Number One Superfood," http://www.westonaprice.org/basicnutrition/codliveroil.html (accessed June 20, 2007).

8. "Durham Research in Primary Schools: The Durham Trial," from the Durham Research Web site at http://durhamtrial.org/primary%20main.htm (accessed June 20, 2007).

9. Jess Halliday, "Nutrition Intervention Trial Looks Promising for SEN Kids," NutraIngredients.com, http://www.nutraingredients.com/news/printNewsBis.asp?id=73281 (accessed June 20, 2007).

10. Bob Greene, M.D., "Diarrhea and Infants," http://www.drgreene.org/body.cfm?id=21&action=detail&ref=581 (accessed June 20, 2007).

Key #3

1. Nicholas Bakalar, "Many Don't Wash Hands After Using the Bathroom," *New York Times*, September 27, 2005, http://www.nytimes.com/2005/09/27/health/27wash.html?ex=1285473600%26en=52f2fbadd9f8c9c8%26ei=5090%26partner=rssuserland%26emc=rss (accessed June 20, 2007).

2. "Britney Barefoot in a Public Bathroom: the German Perspective," Defamer Web site, http://www.defamer.com/topic/britney-barefoot-in-a-public-bathroom-the-german-perspective-020118.php (accessed June 20, 2007).

3. "'Deal or No Deal': Howie's Secret Phobia!", Entertainment Tonight Web site, May 5, 2006, http://www.etonline.com/tv/36354/ (accessed June 20, 2007).

4. Richard Deitsch, "Q&A: Howie Mandel," *Sports Illustrated*, January 29, 2007, 20.

5. Gerald Ensley, "Carting Around More Germs Than Groceries," *Tallahassee Democrat*, 16 January 2005.

6. Carol McGraw, "Cart Attack," *Gazette* (Colorado Springs, CO), December 29, 2005.

7. Ibid.

8. Food Safety Information Council, "Hand Washing Survey: Hand Washing Understanding and Behaviour by Australian Consumers," October 2002, http://www.foodsafety.asn.au/publications/articlesandsurveys/handwashingsurvey.cfm (accessed June 20, 2007).

9. Siri Carpenter, "Modern Hygiene's Dirty Tricks," *Science News* 156, no. 7 (August 14, 1999): 108, http://www.sciencenews.org/pages/pdfs/data/1999/15607/15607-14.pdf (accessed June 20, 2007).

10. German Press Agency, "Do Not Shield Children from Dirt and Illness," *The Raw Story*, October 15, 2006, http://rawstory.com/news/2006/ Do_not_shield_children_from_dirt_an_10152006.html (accessed June 20, 2007).

11. "U.S. Circumcision Rate Drops," Associated Press, June 18, 2007.

12. "Trends in Circumcisions Among Newborns," National Center for Health Statistics, http://www.cdc.gov/nchs/products/pubs/pubd/hestats/circumcisions/circumcisions.htm (accessed July 20, 2007).

13. Edgar J. Schoen et al., "The Highly Protective Effect of Newborn Circumcision Against Invasive Penile Cancer," *Pediatrics* 105, no. 3 (March 2000): e36, http://pediatrics.aappublications.org/cgi/content/full/105/3/e36 (accessed June 20, 2007).

14. "Male Circumcision, Penile Human Papillomavirus Infection, and Cervical Cancer in Female Partners," *The New England Journal of Medicine* (Vol. 346, No. 15: 1105 – 1112).

15. "New Study Shows Benefit of Male Circumcision," American Cancer Society, http://www.cancer.org/docroot/NWS/content/NWS_1_1x_New_Study_Shows_Benefit_ of_Male_Circumcision.asp (accessed July 20, 2007).

16. "Middle Ear Infections," KidsHealth for Parents Web site, http://www.kidshealth.org/ parent/infections/ear/otitis_media.html (accessed June 20, 2007).

17. "Most Ear Infections Host Both Bacteria and Viruses, Study Shows," *ScienceDaily News*, November 7, 2006, and available at http://www.sciencedaily.com/releases/2006/ 11/061106164651.htm (accessed June 20, 2007).

Key #4

1. Greg Botelho, "Roller-Coaster Life of an Indian Icon, Sports' First Star," CNN.com, July 14, 2004, http://edition.cnn.com/2004/WORLD/europe/07/09/jim.thorpe/ (accessed June 20, 2007).

2. Martha Coventry, "Supersizing America," *University of Minnesota News*, Winter 2004, http://www1.umn.edu/umnnews/Feature_Stories/Supersizing_America.html (accessed July 20, 2007).

3. Rich Louv, "Seeing Ourselves in Steve Vaught," *San Diego Union Tribune*, May 9, 2006.

4. Ben Feller, "Some Schools Are Leaving Recess Behind," Associated Press, May 16, 2006, available at http://www.cbsnews.com/stories/2006/05/16/ap/national/mainD8HL5A101.shtml (accessed June 20, 2007).

5. "Banning Recess Boosts Childhood Obesity," Mercola.com, http://www.mercola.com/2006/jul/11/banning_recess_boosts_childhood_obesity.htm (accessed June 20, 2007).

6. "Schools Taking Breaks from Recess," Associated Press, May 15, 2001, and available at http://www.cnnstudentnews.cnn.com/2001/fyi/teachers.ednews/05/15/recess.ap/ (accessed September 2, 2007).

7. Louv, "Seeing Ourselves in Steve Vaught."

8. "Benefits of Rebounding and Bouncercise," American Bio-Compatible Health Systems, Inc., http://www.freedomspring.com/rebounding_benefits.html (accessed July 20, 2007).

9. "National Sleep Foundation 2004 Sleep in America Poll Highlights," http://www.sleepfoundation.org/site/c.huIXKjM0IxF/b.2427941/k.6405/National_Sleep_Foundation_2004_Sleep_in_America_Poll_Highlights.htm (accessed June 20, 2007).

10. Ibid.

11. "Lack of Sleep Causes Obesity," *In the News* newspaper, October 19, 2006.

12. Rong-Gong Lin II, "Sleep, Baby. But . . . Where?", *Los Angeles Times*, September 18, 2006.

13. Stephen Daniells, "Increased Vitamin D May Protect Against Multiple Sclerosis," NutraIngredients Web site, February 20, 2007, http://www.nutraingredients-usa.com/news/ng.asp?id=72919-vitamin-d-multiple-sclerosis-neurological-diseases (accessed June 20, 2007).

14. R. J. Ignelzi, "Taking Cover," *San Diego Union Tribune*, July 4, 2006.

15. Sarah Karnasiewicz, "Do Today's Kids Have 'Nature-Deficit Disorder'?", salon.com, June 2, 2005, http://dir.salon.com/story/mwt/feature/2005/06/02/Louv/index.html?pn=3 (accessed June 20, 2007).

Key #5

1. Centers for Disease Control, "Recommended Immunization Schedules for Persons Aged 0–18 Years —United States, 2007," *MMWR Weekly*, http://www.cdc.gov/mmwr/preview/mmwrhtml/mm5551a7.htm (accessed June 21, 2007), Figure 1.

2. Denise Gellene, "Millions of Women Carry HPV Strains That Vaccine Can Block," *Los Angeles Times*, February 29, 2007, A12.

3. Douglas Fischer, "What's in You?", *Oakland Tribune*, March 18, 2005, and available at http://www.insidebayarea.com/bodyburden/ci_2600879 (accessed June 21, 2007); and Anita Manning, "Autism Disorders Affecting 1 in 150," *USA Today*, February 9, 2007, http://www.usatoday.com/news/health/2007-02-08-autism_x.htm (accessed June 21, 2007).

4. David Ewing Duncan, "The Pollution Within," *National Geographic*, October 2006, 116–43, http://www7.nationalgeographic.com/ngm/0610/feature4/index.html?fs=www3.nationalgeographic.com&fs=plasma.nationalgeographic.com (accessed June 21, 2007).

5. FoodNavigatorUSA, "Microwave Zaps Body Boosting Antioxidants," October 14, 2003, http://www.foodnavigator-usa.com/news/ng.asp?id=47623-microwave-zaps-body (accessed June 21, 2007).

6. Russell Blaylock, M.D., *Excitotoxins: The Taste That Kills* (Santa Fe, New Mexico: Health Press, 1997), 84.

7. Melanie Warner, "The Lowdown on Sweet?", *New York Times*, February 12, 2006, http://www.nytimes.com/2006/02/12/business/yourmoney/12sweet.html?ex=1182571200&en=a319d94d85975efb&ei=5070 (accessed June 21, 2007).

Key #6

1. Paul Pearsall, Ph.D., *The Pleasure Prescription: To Love, to Work, to Play—Life in the Balance* (Alameda, CA: Hunter House, 1996), 63.

2. Gael Crystal and Patrick Flanagan, "Laughter: Still the Best Medicine," 1995, http://www.louienep.com/comedydose/2005/09/laughter_still_the_best_medici.php#more (accessed June 21, 2007).

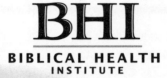

BIBLICAL HEALTH INSTITUTE

The Biblical Health Institute (www.BiblicalHealthInstitute.com) is an online learning community housing educational resources and curricula reinforcing and expanding on Jordan Rubin's Biblical Health message.

Biblical Health Institute provides:

1. "101" level **FREE**, introductory courses corresponding to Jordan's book The Great Physician's Rx for Health and Wellness and its seven keys; Current "101" courses include:

   * "Eating to Live 101"

   * "Whole Food Nutrition Supplements 101"

   * "Advanced Hygiene 101"

   * "Exercise and Body Therapies 101"

   * "Reducing Toxins 101"

   * "Emotional Health 101"

   * "Prayer and Purpose 101"

2. **FREE** resources (healthy recipes, what to E.A.T., resource guide)

3. **FREE** media--videos and video clips of Jordan, music therapy samples, etc.--and much more!

Additionally, Biblical Health Institute also offers in-depth courses for those who want to go deeper.

Course offerings include:

* 40-hour certificate program to become a Biblical Health Coach

* A la carte course offerings designed for personal study and growth (launching late April 2006)

* Home school courses developed by Christian educators, supporting home-schooled students and their parents (designed for middle school and high school ages—launching in August 2006).

For more information and updates on these and other resources go to
www.BiblicalHealthInstitute.com

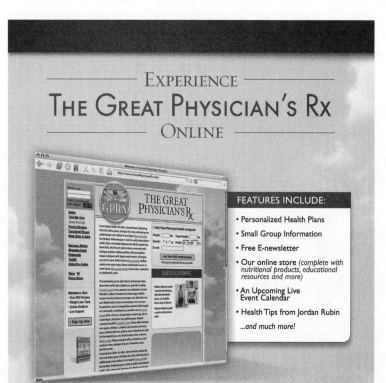

Are you ready to write your own health legacy?

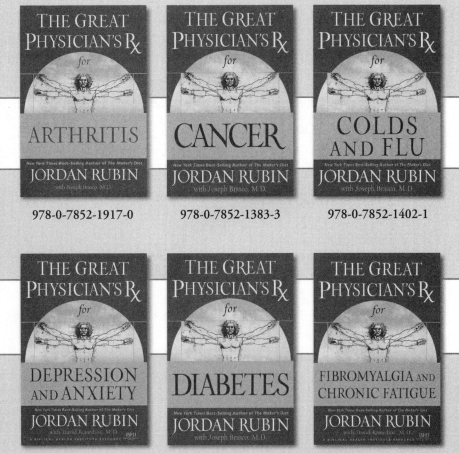

Discover Jordan Rubin's revolutionary plan to wellness in his 12-book Great Physician's Rx series that will transform your health physically, mentally, emotionally, and spiritually.

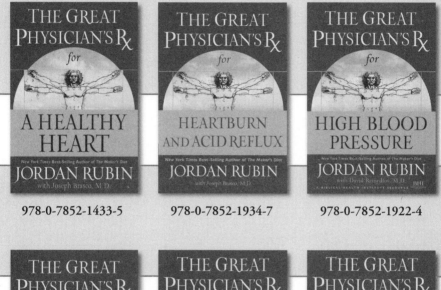
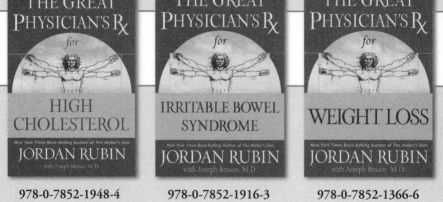
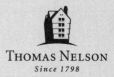